S0-BOK-594

Virtual Clinical Excursions—Medical-Surgical

for

Lewis, Heitkemper, Dirksen, O'Brien, and Bucher: Medical-Surgical Nursing: Assessment and Management of Clinical Problems,

Seventh Edition

prepared by

Dorothy Mathers, RN, MSN
Associate Professor, Nursing
Pennsylvania College of Technology
Williamsport, Pennsylvania

software developed by

Wolfsong Informatics, LLC
Tucson, Arizona

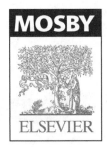

MOSBY

ELSEVIER

MOSBY
ELSEVIER

11830 Westline Industrial Drive
St. Louis, Missouri 63146

VIRTUAL CLINICAL EXCURSIONS—MEDICAL-SURGICAL FOR
LEWIS, HEITKEMPER, DIRKSEN, O'BRIEN, AND BUCHER:
MEDICAL-SURGICAL NURSING: ASSESSMENT AND
MANAGEMENT OF CLINICAL PROBLEMS,
SEVENTH EDITION

ISBN-13: 978-0-323-05014-2
ISBN-10: 0-323-05014-x

Copyright © 2007 by Mosby, Inc., an affiliate of Elsevier Inc.

All rights reserved. No part of this publication may be reproduced or transmitted in any form or by any means, electronic or mechanical, including photocopying, recording, or any information storage and retrieval system, without permission in writing from the publisher. Permissions may be sought directly from Elsevier's Rights Department: phone: (+1) 215 239 3804 (US) or (+44) 1865 843830 (UK); fax: (+44) 1865 853333; e-mail: healthpermissions@elsevier.com. You may also complete your request on-line via the Elsevier website at http://www.elsevier.com/permissions.

Although for mechanical reasons all pages of this publication are perforated, only those pages imprinted with an Elsevier Inc. copyright notice are intended for removal.

Notice

Knowledge and best practice in this field are constantly changing. As new research and experience broaden our knowledge, changes in practice, treatment and drug therapy may become necessary or appropriate. Readers are advised to check the most current information provided (i) on procedures featured or (ii) by the manufacturer of each product to be administered, to verify the recommended dose or formula, the method and duration of administration, and contraindications. It is the responsibility of the practitioner, relying on their own experience and knowledge of the patient, to make diagnoses, to determine dosages and the best treatment for each individual patient, and to take all appropriate safety precautions. To the fullest extent of the law, neither the Publisher nor the Authors assumes any liability for any injury and/or damage to persons or property arising out or related to any use of the material contained in this book.

ISBN-13: 978-0-323-05014-2
ISBN-10: 0-323-05014-x

Executive Editor: *Tom Wilhelm*
Managing Editor: *Jeff Downing*
Associate Developmental Editor: *Tiffany Trautwein*
Book Production Manager: *Gayle May*
Project Manager: *Tracey Schriefer*

Working together to grow
libraries in developing countries

www.elsevier.com | www.bookaid.org | www.sabre.org

ELSEVIER   BOOK AID
            International   Sabre Foundation

Printed in the United States of America

Last digit is the print number: 9 8 7 6 5 4

Workbook
prepared by

Dorothy Mathers, RN, MSN
Associate Professor, Nursing
Pennsylvania College of Technology
Williamsport, Pennsylvania

Textbook

Sharon L. Lewis, RN, PhD, FAAN
Professor, Schools of Nursing and Medicine
Castella Distinguished Professor of Nursing
University of Texas Health Science Center
Clinical Nurse Scientist
Geriatric Research, Education, and Clinical Center
South Texas Veterans Health Care System
San Antonio, Texas

Margaret M. Heitkemper, RN, PhD, FAAN
Professor, Biobehavioral Nursing and Health Systems
School of Nursing
Adjunct Professor, Division of Gastroenterology
School of Medicine
University of Washington
Seattle, Washington

Shannon Ruff Dirksen, RN, PhD
Associate Professor, College of Nursing and Health Care Innovation
Arizona State University
Tempe, Arizona

Patricia Graber O'Brien, APRN BC, BSN, MA, MSN
Instructor, College of Nursing
University of New Mexico
Clinical Research Coordintor, Lovelace Scientific Resources
Albuquerque, New Mexico

Linda Bucher, DSNc, RN
Associate Professor, School of Nursing
University of Delaware
Nursing Research Facilitator, Christiana Care Health System
Newark, Delaware

Reviewers

Peggy Przybycien, RN, MSN
Associate Professor of Nursing
Onondaga Community College
Syracuse, New York

Gina Long, RN, DNSc
Assistant Professor, Department of Nursing
College of Health Professions
Northern Arizona University
Flagstaff, Arizona

Diana Mixon, BSN, MSN
Associate Professor
Department of Nursing
Boise State University
Boise, Idaho

Contents

Unit VIII: Problems of Ingestion, Digestion, Absorption, and Elimination

Unit IX: Problems Related to Regulatory Mechanisms

Unit X: Problems Related to Movement and Coordination

Table of Contents
Lewis, Heitkemper, Dirksen, O'Brien, and Bucher
Medical-Surgical Nursing:
Assessment and Management of Clinical Problems, 7th Edition

Getting Started

GETTING SET UP

■ **MINIMUM SYSTEM REQUIREMENTS**

WINDOWS™

Windows Vista®, XP, 2000 (Recommend Windows XP/2000)
Pentium® III processor (or equivalent) @ 600 MHz (Recommend 800 MHz or better)
256 MB of RAM (Recommend 1 GB or more for Windows Vista®)
800 x 600 screen size (Recommend 1024 x 768)
Thousands of colors
12x CD-ROM drive
Soundblaster 16 soundcard compatibility
Stereo speakers or headphones

Note: Virtual Clinical Excursions—Psychiatric for Windows will require a minimal amount of disk space to install icons and required dll files for Windows 98/ME. Windows Vista® and XP require administrator privileges for installation.

MACINTOSH®

MAC OS X (10.2 or higher)
Apple Power PC G3 @ 500 MHz or better
128 MB of RAM (Recommend 256 MB or more)
800 x 600 screen size (Recommend 1024 x 768)
Thousands of colors
12x CD-ROM drive
Stereo speakers or headphones

Copyright © 2007 by Mosby, Inc., an affiliate of Elsevier Inc. All rights reserved.

■ INSTALLATION INSTRUCTIONS

WINDOWS™

1. Insert the *Virtual Clinical Excursions—Medical-Surgical* CD-ROM.
2. The setup screen should appear automatically if the current product is not already installed. Windows Vista users may be asked to authorize additional security prompts.
3. Follow the onscreen instructions during the setup process.

   If the setup screen does *not* appear automatically (and *Virtual Clinical Excursions—Medical-Surgical* has not been installed already):
   a. Click the **My Computer** icon on your desktop or in your Start menu.
   b. Double-click on your CD-ROM drive.
   c. If installation does not start at this point:
      (1) Click the **Start** icon on the taskbar and select the **Run** option.
      (2) Type d:\setup.exe (where "d:\" is your CD-ROM drive) and press **OK**.
      (3) Follow the onscreen instructions for installation.

MACINTOSH®

1. Insert the *Virtual Clinical Excursions—Medical-Surgical* CD in the CD-ROM drive. The disk icon will appear on your desktop.

2. Double-click on the disk icon.

3. Double-click on the MEDICAL-SURGICAL_MAC run file.

Note: Virtual Clinical Excursions—Medical-Surgical for Macintosh does not have an installation setup and can only be run directly from the CD.

■ HOW TO USE VIRTUAL CLINICAL EXCURSIONS—MEDICAL-SURGICAL

WINDOWS™

1. Double-click on the *Virtual Clinical Excursions—Medical-Surgical* icon located on your desktop.
2. Or navigate to the program via the Windows Start menu.

Note: Windows 98/ME will require you to restart your computer before running the *Virtual Clinical Excursions—Medical-Surgical* program. If your computer uses Windows Vista, right-click on the desktop shortcut and choose Properties. In the Compatability Mode, check the box for "Run as Administrator." Below is a screen capture to show what this looks like.

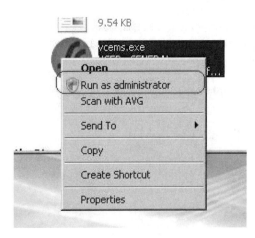

Copyright © 2007 by Mosby, Inc., an affiliate of Elsevier Inc. All rights reserved.

MACINTOSH

1. Insert the *Virtual Clinical Excursions—Medical-Surgical* CD in the CD-ROM drive. The disk icon will appear on your desktop.

2. Double-click on the disk icon.

3. Double-click on the VCEMS_MAC run file.

Note: Virtual Clinical Excursions—Medical-Surgical for Macintosh does not have an installation setup and can only be run directly from the CD.

■ SCREEN SETTINGS

For best results, your computer monitor resolution should be set at a minimum of 800 x 600. The number of colors displayed should be set to "thousands or higher" (High Color or 16 bit) or "millions of colors" (True Color or 24 bit).

Windows

1. From the **Start** menu, select **Control Panel** (on some systems, you will first go to **Settings**, then to **Control Panel**).
2. Double-click on the **Display** icon.
3. Click on the **Settings** tab.
4. Under **Screen resolution** use the slider bar to select **800 by 600 pixels**.
5. Access the **Colors** drop-down menu by clicking on the down arrow.
6. Select **High Color (16 bit)** or **True Color (24 bit)**.
7. Click on **OK**.
8. You may be asked to verify the setting changes. Click **Yes**.
9. You may be asked to restart your computer to accept the changes. Click **Yes**.

Macintosh

1. Select the **Monitors** control panel.
2. Select **800 x 600** (or similar) from the **Resolution** area.
3. Select **Thousands** or **Millions** from the **Color Depth** area.

■ WEB BROWSERS

Supported web browsers include Microsoft Internet Explorer (IE) version 6.0 or higher and Mozilla Firefox version 2.0 or higher. The supported browser for Macs running OS X is Mozilla Firefox.

If you use America Online® (AOL) for web access, you will need AOL version 4.0 or higher and one of the browsers listed above. Do not use earlier versions of AOL with earlier versions of IE, because you will have difficulty accessing many features.

For best results with AOL:
• Connect to the Internet using AOL version 4.0 or higher.
• Open a private chat within AOL (this allows the AOL client to remain open, without asking whether you wish to disconnect while minimized).
• Minimize AOL.
• Launch a recommended browser.

Copyright © 2007 by Mosby, Inc., an affiliate of Elsevier Inc. All rights reserved.

■ TECHNICAL SUPPORT

Technical support for this product is available between 7:30 a.m. and 7 p.m. (CST), Monday through Friday. Before calling, be sure that your computer meets the minimum system requirements to run this software. Inside the United States and Canada, call 1-800-692-9010. Outside North America, call 314-872-8370. You may also fax your questions to 314-523-4932 or contact Technical Support through e-mail: technical.support@elsevier.com.

Trademarks: Windows, Macintosh, Pentium, and America Online are registered trademarks.

Copyright © 2007 by Mosby, Inc., an affiliate of Elsevier Inc.

All rights reserved. No part of this product may be reproduced or transmitted in any form or by any means, electronic or mechanical, including input or storage in any information system, without written permission from the publisher.

ACCESSING *Virtual Clinical Excursions—Medical-Surgical* FROM EVOLVE

The product you have purchased is part of the Evolve family of online courses and learning resources. Please read the following information thoroughly to get started.

To access your instructor's course on Evolve:

Your instructor will provide you with the username and password needed to access this specific course on the Evolve Learning System. Once you have received this information, please follow these instructions:

1. Go to the Evolve student page (http://evolve.elsevier.com/student)

2. Enter your username and password in the **Login to My Evolve** area and click the **Login** button.

3. You will be taken to your personalized **My Evolve** page, where the course will be listed in the **My Courses** module.

TECHNICAL REQUIREMENTS

To use an Evolve course, you will need access to a computer that is connected to the Internet and equipped with web browser software that supports frames. For optimal performance, it is recommended that you have speakers and use a high-speed Internet connection. However, slower dial-up modems (56 K minimum) are acceptable.

Copyright © 2007 by Mosby, Inc., an affiliate of Elsevier Inc. All rights reserved.

Whichever browser you use, the browser preferences must be set to enable cookies and JavaScript and the cache must be set to reload every time.

Enable Cookies

Browser	Steps
Internet Explorer (IE) 6.0 or higher	1. Select **Tools → Internet Options**. 2. Select **Privacy** tab. 3. Use the slider (slide down) to **Accept All Cookies**. 4. Click **OK**. -OR- 3. Click the **Advanced** button. 4. Click the check box next to **Override Automatic Cookie Handling**. 5. Click the **Accept** radio buttons under **First-party Cookies** and **Third-party Cookies**. 6. Click **OK**.
Mozilla Firefox 2.0 or higher	1. Select **Tools → Options**. 2. Select the **Privacy** icon. 3. Click to expand Cookies. 4. Select **Allow sites to set cookies**. 5. Click **OK**.

Set Cache to Always Reload a Page

Browser	Steps
Internet Explorer (IE) 6.0 or higher	1. Select **Tools → Internet Options**. 2. Select **General** tab. 3. Go to the **Temporary Internet Files** and click the **Settings** button. 4. Select the radio button for **Every visit to the page** and click **OK** when complete.
Mozilla Firefox 2.0 or higher	1. Select **Tools → Options**. 2. Select the **Privacy** icon. 3. Click to expand Cache. 4. Set the value to "**0**" in the **Use up to: __ MB of disk space for the cache** field. 5. Click **OK**.

Copyright © 2007 by Mosby, Inc., an affiliate of Elsevier Inc. All rights reserved.

Enable JavaScript

Browser	Steps
Internet Explorer (IE) 6.0 or higher	1. Select **Tools → Internet Options**. 2. Select **Security** tab. 3. Under **Security level for this zone** set to **Medium** or lower.
Netscape 7.1 or higher	1. Select **Edit → Preferences**. 2. Select **Advanced**. 3. Select **Scripts & Plugins**. 4. Make sure the **Navigator** box is checked to **Enable JavaScript**. 5. Click **OK**.
Mozilla Firefox 1.4 or higher	1. Select **Tools → Options**. 2. Select the **Content** icon. 3. Select **Enable JavaScript**. 4. Click **OK**.

Set Cache to Always Reload a Page

Browser	Steps
Internet Explorer (IE) 6.0 or higher	1. Select **Tools → Internet Options**. 2. Select **General** tab. 3. Go to the **Temporary Internet Files** and click the **Settings** button. 4. Select the radio button for **Every visit to the page** and click **OK** when complete.
Netscape 7.1 or higher	1. Select **Edit → Preferences**. 2. Select **Advanced**. 3. Select **Cache**. 4. Select the **Every time I view the page** radio button. 5. Click **OK**.
Mozilla Firefox 1.4 or higher	1. Select **Tools → Options**. 2. Select the **Privacy** icon. 3. Click to expand Cache. 4. Set the value to "**0**" in the **Use up to: ___ MB of disk space for the cache** field. 5. Click **OK**.

Copyright © 2007 by Mosby, Inc., an affiliate of Elsevier Inc. All rights reserved.

<u>Plug-Ins</u>

Adobe Acrobat Reader—With the free Acrobat Reader software, you can view and print Adobe PDF files. Many Evolve products offer student and instructor manuals, checklists, and more in this format!

Download at: http://www.adobe.com

Apple QuickTime—Install this to hear word pronunciations, heart and lung sounds, and many other helpful audio clips within Evolve Online Courses!

Download at: http://www.apple.com

Adobe Flash Player—This player will enhance your viewing of many Evolve web pages, as well as educational short-form to long-form animation within the Evolve Learning System!

Download at: http://www.adobe.com

Adobe Shockwave Player—Shockwave is best for viewing the many interactive learning activities within Evolve Online Courses!

Download at: http://www.adobe.com

Microsoft Word Viewer—With this viewer Microsoft Word users can share documents with those who don't have Word, and users without Word can open and view Word documents. Many Evolve products have testbank, student and instructor manuals, and other documents available for downloading and viewing on your own computer!

Download at: http://www.microsoft.com

Microsoft PowerPoint Viewer—View PowerPoint 97, 2000, and 2002 presentations even if you don't have PowerPoint with this viewer. Many Evolve products have slides available for downloading and viewing on your own computer!

Download at: http://www.microsoft.com

Copyright © 2007 by Mosby, Inc., an affiliate of Elsevier Inc. All rights reserved.

SUPPORT INFORMATION

Live support is available to customers in the United States and Canada from 7:30 a.m. to 7 p.m. (CST), Monday through Friday by calling **1-800-401-9962**. You can also send an email to evolve-support@elsevier.com.

There is also **24/7 support information** available on the Evolve website (http://evolve.elsevier.com), including:

- Guided Tours
- Tutorials
- Frequently Asked Questions (FAQs)
- Online Copies of Course User Guides
- And much more!

Copyright © 2007 by Mosby, Inc., an affiliate of Elsevier Inc. All rights reserved.

A QUICK TOUR

Welcome to *Virtual Clinical Excursions—Medical-Surgical*, a virtual hospital setting in which you can work with multiple complex patient simulations and also learn to access and evaluate the information resources that are essential for high-quality patient care.

The virtual hospital, Pacific View Regional Hospital, has realistic architecture and access to patient rooms, a Nurses' Station, and a Medication Room.

■ BEFORE YOU START

Make sure you have your textbook nearby when you use the *Virtual Clinical Excursions—Medical-Surgical* CD. You will want to consult topic areas in your textbook frequently while working with the CD and using this workbook.

■ HOW TO SIGN IN

- Enter your name on the Student Nurse identification badge.
- Now choose one of the four periods of care in which to work. In Periods of Care 1 through 3, you can actively engage in patient assessment, entry of data in the electronic patient record (EPR), and medication administration. Period of Care 4 presents the day in review. Highlight and click the appropriate period of care. (For this quick tour, choose **Period of Care 1: 0730-0815**.)
- This takes you to the Patient List screen (see example on page 11). Only the patients on the Medical-Surgical Floor are available. Note that the virtual time is provided in the box at the lower left corner of the screen (0730, since we chose Period of Care 1).

Note: If you choose to work during Period of Care 4: 1900-2000, the Patient List screen is skipped since you are not able to visit patients or administer medications during the shift. Instead, you are taken directly to the Nurses' Station, where the records of all the patients on the floor are available for your review.

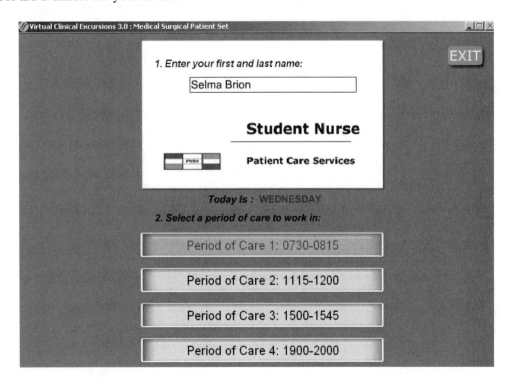

Copyright © 2007 by Mosby, Inc., an affiliate of Elsevier Inc. All rights reserved.

■ **PATIENT LIST**

MEDICAL-SURGICAL UNIT

Harry George (Room 401)
Osteomyelitis—A 54-year-old Caucasian male admitted from a homeless shelter with an infected leg. He has complications of type 2 diabetes mellitus, alcohol abuse, nicotine addiction, poor pain control, and complex psychosocial issues.

Jacquline Catanazaro (Room 402)
Asthma—A 45-year-old Caucasian female admitted with an acute asthma exacerbation and suspected pneumonia. She has complications of chronic schizophrenia, noncompliance with medication therapy, obesity, and herniated disk.

Piya Jordan (Room 403)
Bowel obstruction—A 68-year-old Asian female admitted with a colon mass and suspected adenocarcinoma. She undergoes a right hemicolectomy. This patient's complications include atrial fibrillation, hypokalemia, and symptoms of meperidine toxicity.

Clarence Hughes (Room 404)
Degenerative joint disease—A 73-year-old African-American male admitted for a left total knee replacement. His preparations for discharge are complicated by the development of a pulmonary embolus and the need for ongoing intravenous therapy.

Pablo Rodriguez (Room 405)
Metastatic lung carcinoma—A 71-year-old Hispanic male admitted with symptoms of dehydration and malnutrition. He has chronic pain secondary to multiple subcutaneous skin nodules and psychosocial concerns related to family issues with his approaching death.

Patricia Newman (Room 406)
Pneumonia—A 61-year-old Caucasian female admitted with worsening pulmonary function and an acute respiratory infection. Her chronic emphysema is complicated by heavy smoking, hypertension, and malnutrition. She needs access to community resources such as a smoking cessation program and meal assistance.

Copyright © 2007 by Mosby, Inc., an affiliate of Elsevier Inc. All rights reserved.

■ HOW TO SELECT A PATIENT

- You can choose one or more patients to work with from the Patient List by checking the box to the left of the patient name(s). For this quick tour, select Piya Jordan and Pablo Rodriguez. (In order to receive a scorecard for a patient, the patient must be selected before proceeding to the Nurses' Station.)
- Click on **Get Report** to the right of the medical records number (MRN) to view a summary of the patient's care during the 12-hour period before your arrival on the unit.
- After reviewing the report, click on **Return to Patient List** and repeat the previous step to review the report of your second patient.
- When you are ready to begin your care, click on **Go to Nurses' Station** in the right lower corner.

Note: Even though the Patient List is initially skipped when you sign in to work for Period of Care 4, you can still access this screen if you wish to review the shift-change report for any of the patients. To do so, simply click on **Patient List** near the top left corner of the Nurses' Station (or click on the clipboard to the left of the Kardex). Then click on **Get Report** for the patient(s) whose care you are reviewing. This may be done during any period of care.

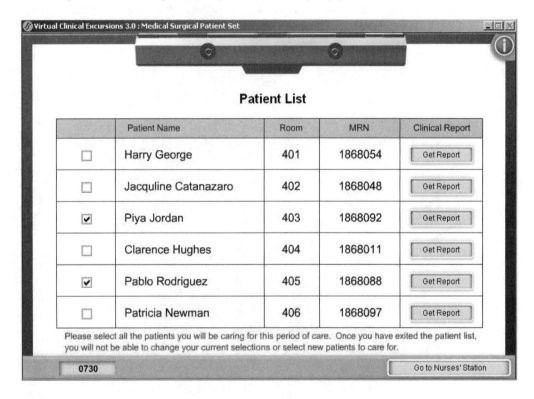

Copyright © 2007 by Mosby, Inc., an affiliate of Elsevier Inc. All rights reserved.

■ HOW TO FIND A PATIENT'S RECORDS

NURSES' STATION

Within the Nurses' Station, you will see:

1. A clipboard that contains the patient list for that floor.
2. A chart rack with patient charts labeled by room number, a notebook labeled Kardex, and a notebook labeled MAR (Medication Administration Record).
3. A desktop computer with access to the Electronic Patient Record (EPR).
4. A tool bar across the top of the screen that can also be used to access the Patient List, EPR, Chart, MAR, and Kardex. This tool bar is also accessible from each patient's room.
5. A Drug Guide containing information about the medications you are able to administer to your patients.
6. A tool bar across the bottom of the screen that you can use to access patient rooms, the Medication Room, the Floor Map, or the Drug Guide.

As you run your cursor over an item, it will be highlighted. To select, simply double-click on the item. As you use these resources, you will always be able to return to the Nurses' Station by clicking on the **Return to Nurses' Station** bar located in the right lower corner of your screen.

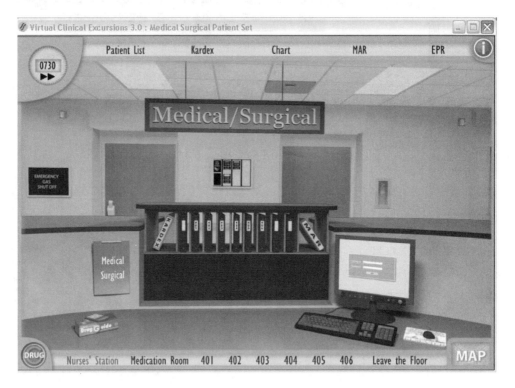

Copyright © 2007 by Mosby, Inc., an affiliate of Elsevier Inc. All rights reserved.

MEDICATION ADMINISTRATION RECORD (MAR)

The MAR icon located in the tool bar at the top of your screen accesses current 24-hour medications for each patient. Click on the icon and the MAR will open. (*Note:* You can also access the MAR by clicking on the MAR notebook on the far right side of the book rack in the center of the screen.) Within the MAR, tabs on the right side of the screen allow you to select patients by room number. Be careful to make sure you select the correct tab number for *your* patient rather than simply reading the first record that appears after the MAR opens. Each MAR sheet lists the following:

- Medications
- Route and dosage of each medication
- Times of administration of each medication

Note: The MAR changes each day. Expired MARs are stored in the patients' charts.

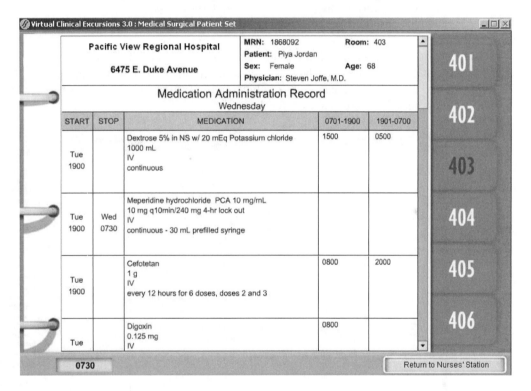

Copyright © 2007 by Mosby, Inc., an affiliate of Elsevier Inc. All rights reserved.

CHARTS

To access patient charts, either click on the **Chart** icon at the top of your screen or anywhere within the chart rack in the center of the Nurses' Station screen. When the close-up view appears, the individual charts are labeled by room number. To open a chart, click on the room number of the patient whose chart you wish to review. The patient's name and allergies will appear on the left side of the screen, along with a list of tabs on the right side of the screen, allowing you to view the following data:

- Allergies
- Physician's Orders
- Physician's Notes
- Nurse's Notes
- Laboratory Reports
- Diagnostic Reports
- Surgical Reports
- Consultations
- Patient Education
- History and Physical
- Nursing Admission
- Expired MARs
- Consents
- Mental Health
- Admissions
- Emergency Department

Information appears in real time. The entries are in reverse chronologic order, so use the down arrow at the right side of each chart page to scroll down to view previous entries. Flip from tab to tab to view multiple data fields or click on the **Return to Nurses' Station** bar in the lower right corner of the screen to exit the chart.

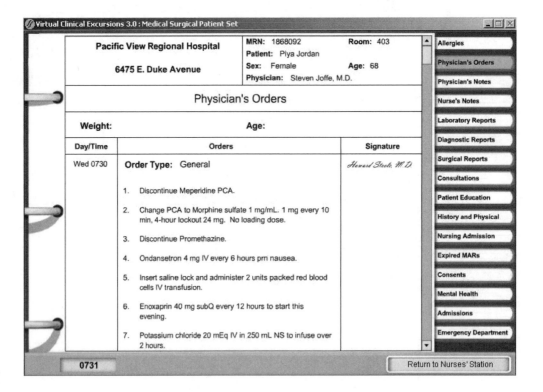

Copyright © 2007 by Mosby, Inc., an affiliate of Elsevier Inc. All rights reserved.

ELECTRONIC PATIENT RECORD (EPR)

The EPR can be accessed from the computer in the Nurses' Station or from the EPR icon located in the tool bar at the top of your screen. To access a patient's EPR:

- Click on either the computer screen or the **EPR** icon.
- Your username and password are automatically filled in.
- Click on **Login** to enter the EPR.
- *Note:* Like the MAR, the EPR is arranged numerically. Thus when you enter, you are initially shown the records of the patient in the lowest room number on the floor. To view the correct data for *your* patient, remember to select the correct room number, using the drop-down menu for the Patient field at the top left corner of the screen.

The EPR used in Pacific View Regional Hospital represents a composite of commercial versions being used in hospitals. You can access the EPR:

- to review existing data for a patient (by room number).
- to enter data you collect while working with a patient.

The EPR is updated daily, so no matter what day or part of a shift you are working, there will be a current EPR with the patient's data from the past days of the current hospital stay. This type of simulated EPR allows you to examine how data for different attributes have changed over time, as well as to examine data for all of a patient's attributes at a particular time. The EPR is fully functional (as it is in a real-life hospital). You can enter such data as blood pressure, breath sounds, and certain treatments. The EPR will not, however, allow you to enter data for a previous time period. Use the arrows at the bottom of the screen to move forward and backward in time.

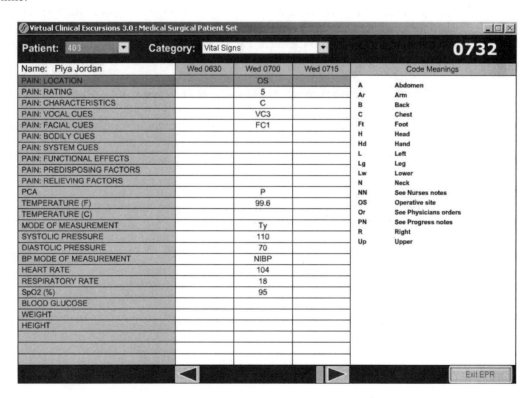

Copyright © 2007 by Mosby, Inc., an affiliate of Elsevier Inc. All rights reserved.

At the top of the EPR screen, you can choose patients by their room numbers. In addition, you have access to 17 different categories of patient data. To change patients or data categories, click the down arrow to the right of the room number or category.

The categories of patient data in the EPR as as follows:

- Vital Signs
- Respiratory
- Cardiovascular
- Neurologic
- Gastrointestinal
- Excretory
- Musculoskeletal
- Integumentary
- Reproductive
- Psychosocial
- Wounds and Drains
- Activity
- Hygiene and Comfort
- Safety
- Nutrition
- IV
- Intake and Output

Remember, each hospital selects its own codes. The codes used in the EPR at Pacific View Regional Hospital may be different from ones you have seen in your clinical rotations. Take some time to acquaint yourself with the codes. Within the Vital Signs category, click on any item in the left column (e.g., Pain: Characteristics). In the far-right column, you will see a list of code meanings for the possible findings and/or descriptors for that assessment area.

You will use the codes to record the data you collect as you work with patients. Click on the box in the last time column to the right of any item and wait for the code meanings applicable to that entry to appear. Select the appropriate code to describe your assessment findings and type it in the box. (*Note:* If no cursor appears within the box, click on the box again until the blue shading disappears and the blinking cursor appears.) Once the data are typed in this box, they are entered into the patient's record for this period of care only.

To leave the EPR, click on **Exit EPR** in the bottom right corner of the screen.

Copyright © 2007 by Mosby, Inc., an affiliate of Elsevier Inc. All rights reserved.

■ **VISITING A PATIENT**

From the Nurses' Station, click on the room number of the patient you wish to visit in the tool bar at the bottom of your screen. Once you are inside the room, you will see a still photo of your patient in the top left corner. To verify that this is the patient you have chosen, click on the **Check Armband** icon to the right of the photo. The patient's identification data will appear. If you click on **Check Allergies** (the next icon to the right), a list of the patient's allergies (if any) will replace the photo.

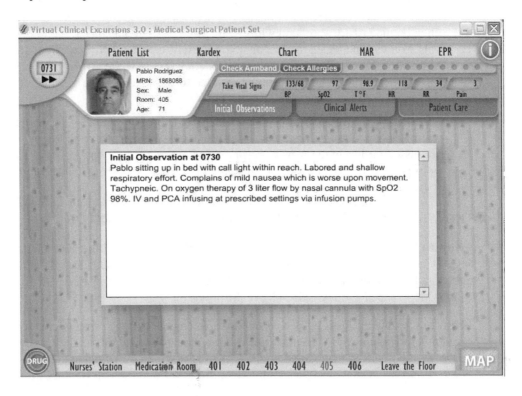

Also located in the patient's room are multiple icons you can use to assess the patient or the patient's medications. A virtual clock is provided in the upper left corner of the room to monitor your progress in real time. (*Note:* The fast-forward icon within the virtual clock will advance the time by 2-minute intervals when clicked.)

- The tool bar across the top of the screen allows you to check the **Patient List**, access the **EPR** to check or enter data, and view the patient's **Chart**, **MAR**, or **Kardex**.

- The **Take Vital Signs** icon allows you to measure the patient's up-to-the-minute blood pressure, oxygen saturation, temperature, heart rate, respiratory rate, and pain level.

- Each time you enter a patient's room, you are given an Initial Observation report to review (in the text box under the patient's photo). These notes are provided to give you a "look" at the patient as if you had just stepped into the room. You can also click on the **Initial Observations** icon to return to this box from other views within the patient's room. To the right of this icon is **Clinical Alerts**, a resource that allows you to make decisions about priority medication interventions based on emerging data collected in real time. Check this screen throughout your period of care to avoid missing critical information related to recently ordered or STAT medications.

- Clicking on the **Patient Care** icon opens up three specific learning environments within the patient room: **Physical Assessment**, **Nurse-Client Interactions**, and **Medication Administration**.

- To perform a **Physical Assessment**, choose a body area (such as **Head & Neck**) by clicking on the appropriate icon in the column of yellow buttons. This activates a list of system subcategories for that body area (e.g., see **Sensory**, **Neurologic**, etc. in the green boxes). After

Copyright © 2007 by Mosby, Inc., an affiliate of Elsevier Inc. All rights reserved.

you click on the system that you wish to evaluate, a still photo and text box appear, describing the assessment findings. The still photo is a "snapshot" of how an assessment of this area might be done or what the finding might look like. For every body area, there is also an **Equipment** button located on the far right of the screen.

• To the right of the Physical Assessment icon is **Nurse-Client Interactions**. Clicking on this icon will reveal the times and titles of any videos available for viewing. (*Note:* If the video you wish to see is not listed, this means you have not yet reached the correct virtual time to view that video. Check the virtual clock; you may return to access the video once its designated time has occurred—as long as you do so within the same period of care. Or you can click on the fast-forward icon within the virtual clock to advance the time by 2-minute intervals. You will then need to click again on **Patient Care** and **Nurse-Client Interactions** to refresh the screen.) To view a listed video, click on the white arrow to the right of the video title. Use the control buttons below the video to start, stop, pause, rewind, or fast-forward the action or to mute the sound.

• **Medication Administration** is the pathway that allows you to review and administer medications to a patient after you have prepared them in the Medication Room. This process is addressed further in the *How to Prepare Medications* section (pages 19-20) and in *Medications* (pages 26-30). For additional hands-on practice, see *Reducing Medication Errors* (pages 37-41).

■ HOW TO QUIT, CHANGE PATIENTS, OR CHANGE PERIOD OF CARE

How to Quit: From most screens, you may click the **Leave the Floor** icon on the bottom tool bar to the right of the patient room numbers. (*Note:* From some screens, you will first need to click an **Exit** button or **Return to Nurses' Station** before clicking **Leave the Floor**.) When the Floor Menu appears, click **Exit** to leave the program.

How to Change Patients or Period of Care: To change patients, simply click on the new patient's room number. (You cannot receive a scorecard for a new patient, however, unless you have already selected that patient on the Patient List screen.) To change to a new period of care or to restart the virtual clock, click on **Leave the Floor** and then on **Restart the Program**.

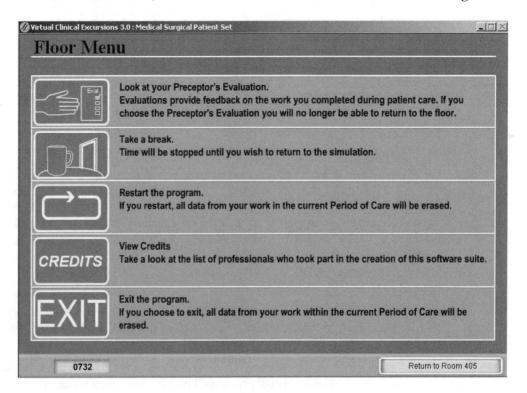

Copyright © 2007 by Mosby, Inc., an affiliate of Elsevier Inc. All rights reserved.

■ HOW TO PREPARE MEDICATIONS

From the Nurses' Station or the patient's room, you can access the Medication Room by clicking on the icon in the tool bar at the bottom of your screen to the left of the patient room numbers.

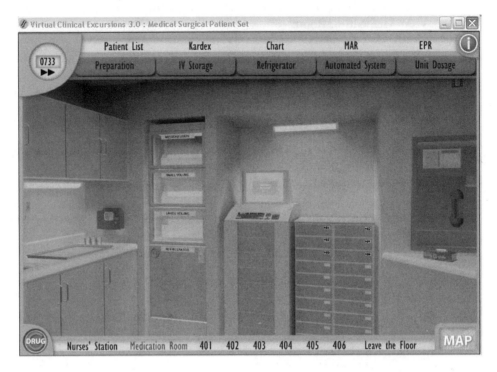

In the Medication Room you have access to the following (from left to right):

- A preparation area is located on the counter under the cabinets. To begin the medication preparation process, click on the tray on the counter or click on the **Preparation** icon at the top of the screen. The next screen leads you through a specific sequence (called the Preparation Wizard) to prepare medications one at a time for administration to a patient. However, no medication has been selected at this time. We will do this while working with a patient in *A Detailed Tour*. To exit this screen, click on **View Medication Room**.

- To the right of the cabinets (and above the refrigerator), IV storage bins are provided. Click on the bins themselves or on the **IV Storage** icon at the top of the screen. The bins are labeled **Microinfusion, Small Volume**, and **Large Volume**. Click on an individual bin to see a list of its contents. If you needed to prepare an IV medication at this time, you could click on the medication and its label would appear to the right under the patient's name. Next, you would click **Put Medication on Tray**. If you ever change your mind or choose the incorrect medication, you can reverse your actions by clicking on **Put Medication in Bin**. Click **Close Bin** in the right bottom corner to exit. **View Medication Room** brings you back to a full view of the entire room.

- A refrigerator is located under the IV storage bins to hold any medications that must be stored below room temperature. Click on the refrigerator door or on the **Refrigerator** icon at the top of the screen. Then click on the close-up view of the door to access the medications. When you are finished, click **Close Door** and then **View Medication Room**.

Copyright © 2007 by Mosby, Inc., an affiliate of Elsevier Inc. All rights reserved.

- To prepare controlled substances, click the **Automated System** icon at the top of the screen or click the computer monitor located to the right of the IV storage bins. A login screen will appear; your name and password are automatically filled in. Click **Login**. Select the patient for whom you wish to access medications; then select the correct medication drawer to open (they are stored alphabetically). Click **Open Drawer**, highlight the proper medication, and choose **Put Medication on Tray**. When you are finished, click **Close Drawer** and then **View Medication Room**.

- Next to the Automated System is a set of drawers identified by patient room number. To access these, click on the drawers themselves or on the **Unit Dosage** icon at the top of the screen. This provides a close-up view of the drawers. To open a drawer, click on the room number of the patient you are working with. Next, click on the medication you would like to prepare for the patient, and a label will appear to the right, listing the medication strength, units, and dosage per unit. You can **Open** and **Close** this medication label by clicking the appropriate icon. To exit, click **Close Drawer**; then click **View Medication Room**.

At any time, you can learn about a medication you wish to prepare for a patient by clicking on the **Drug** icon in the bottom left corner of the medication room screen or by clicking the **Drug Guide** book on the counter to the right of the unit dosage drawers. The **Drug Guide** provides information about the medications commonly included in nursing drug handbooks. Nutritional supplements and maintenance intravenous fluid preparations are not included.

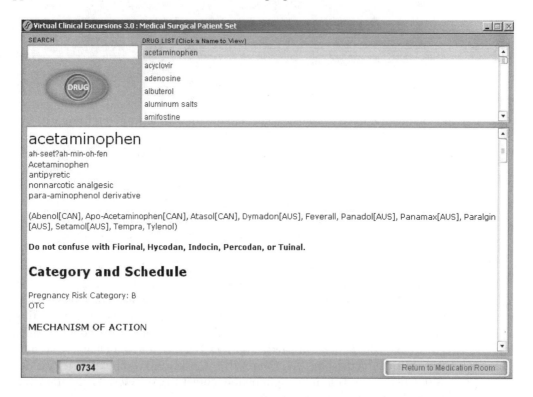

To access the MAR to review the medications ordered for a patient, click on the **MAR** icon located in the tool bar at the top of your screen and then click on the correct tab for your patient's room number. You may also click the **Review MAR** icon in the tool bar at the bottom of your screen from inside each medication storage area.

After you have chosen and prepared your medications, return to the patient's room to administer them by clicking on the room number in the bottom tool bar. Once inside the patient's room, click on **Patient Care** and then on **Medication Administration** and follow the proper administration sequence.

Copyright © 2007 by Mosby, Inc., an affiliate of Elsevier Inc. All rights reserved.

■ PRECEPTOR'S EVALUATIONS

When you have finished a session, click on **Leave the Floor** to go to the Floor Menu. At this point, you can click on the top icon (**Look at Your Preceptor's Evaluation**) to receive a score-card that provides feedback on the work you completed during patient care.

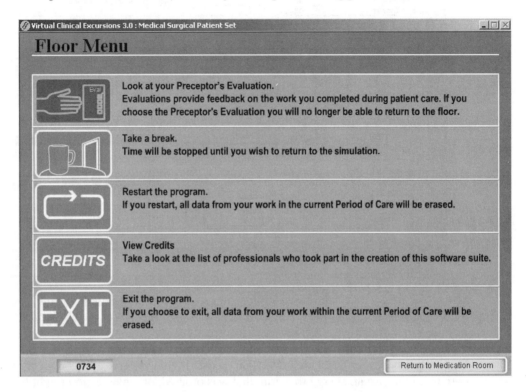

Evaluations are available for each patient you selected when you signed in for the current period of care. Click on the **Medication Scorecard** icon to see an example.

Copyright © 2007 by Mosby, Inc., an affiliate of Elsevier Inc. All rights reserved.

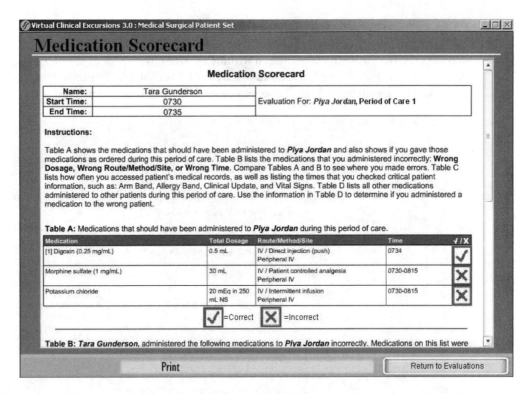

The scorecard compares the medications you administered to a patient during a period of care with what should have been administered. Table A lists the correct medications. Table B lists any medications that were administered incorrectly.

Remember, not every medication listed on the MAR should necessarily be given. For example, a patient might have an allergy to a drug that was ordered, or a medication might have been improperly transcribed to the MAR. Predetermined medication "errors" embedded within the program challenge you to exercise critical thinking skills and professional judgment when deciding to administer a medication, just as you would in a real hospital. Use all your available resources, such as the patient's chart and the MAR, to make your decision.

Table C lists the resources that were available to assist you in medication administration. It also documents whether and when you accessed these resources. For example, did you check the patient armband or perform a check of vital signs? If so, when?

You can click **Print** to get a copy of this report if needed. When you have finished reviewing the scorecard, click **Return to Evaluations** and then **Return to Menu**.

Copyright © 2007 by Mosby, Inc., an affiliate of Elsevier Inc. All rights reserved.

■ FLOOR MAP

To get a general sense of your location within the hospital, you can click on the **Map** icon found in the lower right corner of most of the screens in the *Virtual Clinical Excursions—Medical-Surgical* program. (*Note:* If you are following this quick tour step by step, you will need to **Restart the Program** from the Floor Menu, sign in again, and go to the Nurses' Station to access the map.) When you click the **Map** icon, a floor map appears, showing the layout of the floor you are currently on, as well as a directory of the patients and services on that floor. As you move your cursor over the directory list, the location of each room is highlighted on the map (and vice versa). The floor map can be accessed from the Nurses' Station, Medication Room, and each patient's room.

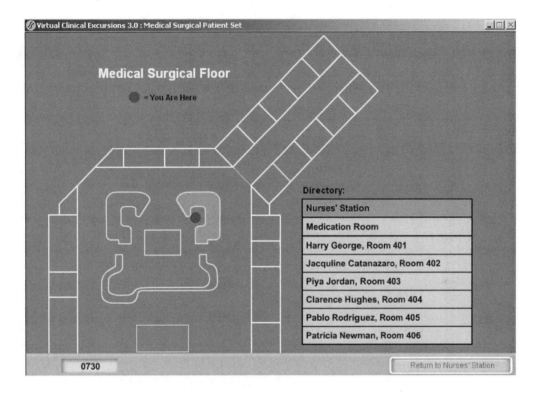

Copyright © 2007 by Mosby, Inc., an affiliate of Elsevier Inc. All rights reserved.

A DETAILED TOUR

If you wish to more thoroughly understand the capabilities of *Virtual Clinical Excursions—Medical-Surgical*, take a detailed tour by completing the following section. During this tour, we will work with a specific patient to introduce you to all the different components and learning opportunities available within the software.

■ WORKING WITH A PATIENT

Sign in for Period of Care 1 (0730-0815). From the Patient List, select Piya Jordan in Room 403; however, do not go to the Nurses' Station yet.

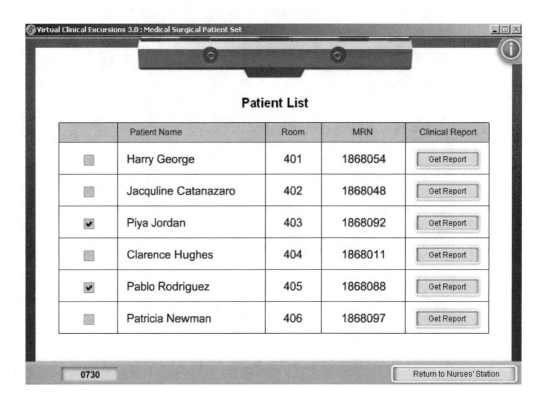

■ REPORT

In hospitals, when one shift ends and another begins, the outgoing nurse who attended a patient will give a verbal and sometimes a written summary of that patient's condition to the incoming nurse who will assume care for the patient. This summary is called a report and is an important source of data to provide an overview of a patient. Your first task is to get the clinical report on Piya Jordan. To do this, click **Get Report** in the far right column in this patient's row. From a brief review of this summary, identify the problems and areas of concern that you will need to address for this patient.

When you have finished noting any areas of concern, click **Go to Nurses' Station**.

Copyright © 2007 by Mosby, Inc., an affiliate of Elsevier Inc. All rights reserved.

■ CHARTS

You can access Piya Jordan's chart from the Nurses' Station or from the patient's room (403). We will access it from the Nurses' Station: Click on the chart rack or on the **Chart** icon in the tool bar at the top of your screen. Next, click on the chart labeled **403** to open the medical record for Piya Jordan. Click on the **Emergency Department** tab to view a record of why this patient was admitted.

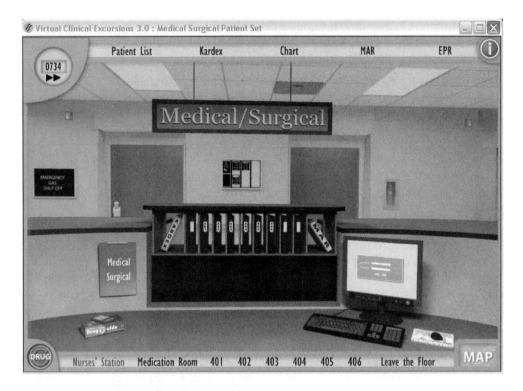

How many days has Piya Jordan been in the hospital?

What tests were done upon her arrival in the Emergency Department and why?

What was her reason for admission?

You should also click on **Surgical Reports** to learn what procedures were performed and when. Finally, review the **Nursing Admission** and **History and Physical** to learn about the health history of this patient. When you are done reviewing the chart, click **Return to Nurses' Station**.

Copyright © 2007 by Mosby, Inc., an affiliate of Elsevier Inc. All rights reserved.

■ MEDICATIONS

Open the Medication Administration Record (MAR) by clicking on the **MAR** icon in the tool bar at the top of your screen. *Remember:* The MAR automatically opens to the first occupied room number on the floor—which is not necessarily your patient's room number! Since you need to access Piya Jordan's MAR, click on tab **403** (her room number). Always make sure you are giving the *Right Drug to the Right Patient!*

Examine the list of medications ordered for Piya Jordan. In the table below, list the medications that need to be given during this period of care (0730-0815). For each medication, note the dosage, route, and time to be given.

Time	Medication	Dosage	Route

Click on **Return to Nurses' Station**. Next, click on **403** on the bottom tool bar and then verify that you are indeed in Piya Jordan's room. Select **Clinical Alerts** (the icon to the right of Initial Observations) to check for any emerging data that might affect your medication administration priorities. Next, go to the patient's chart (click on the **Chart** icon; then click on **403**). When the chart opens, select the **Physician's Orders** tab.

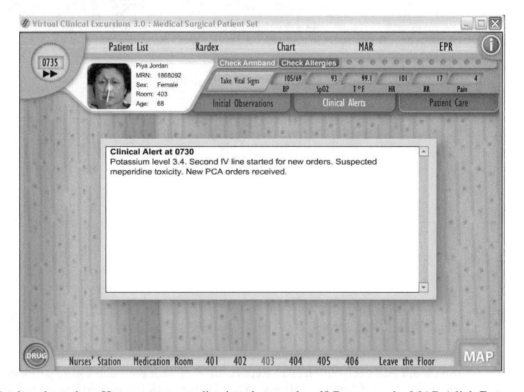

Review the orders. Have any new medications been ordered? Return to the MAR (click **Return to Room 403**; then click **MAR**). Verify that the new medications have been correctly transcribed to the MAR. Mistakes are sometimes made in the transcription process in the hospital setting, and it is sound practice to double-check any new order.

Copyright © 2007 by Mosby, Inc., an affiliate of Elsevier Inc. All rights reserved.

Are there any patient assessments you will need to perform before administering these medications? If so, return to Room 403 and click on **Patient Care** and then **Physical Assessment** to complete those assessments before proceeding.

Now click on the **Medication Room** icon in the tool bar at the bottom of your screen to locate and prepare the medications for Piya Jordan.

In the Medication Room, you must access the medications for Piya Jordan from the specific dispensing system in which each medication is stored. Locate each medication that needs to be given in this time period and click on **Put Medication on Tray** as appropriate. (*Hint:* Look in Unit Dosage drawer first.) When you are finished, click on **Close Drawer** and then on **View Medication Room**. Now click on the medication tray on the counter on the left side of the medication room screen to begin preparing the medications you have selected. (*Remember:* You can also click **Preparation** in the tool bar at the top of the screen.)

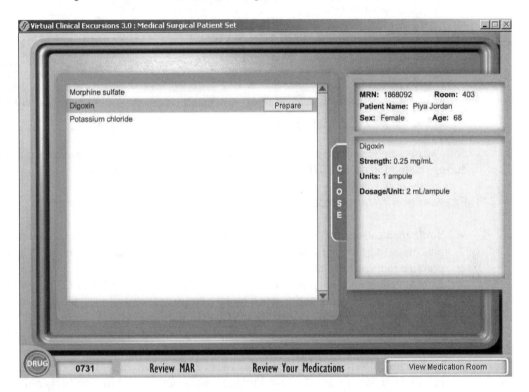

In the preparation area, you should see a list of the medications you put on the tray in the previous steps. Click on the first medication and then click **Prepare**. Follow the onscreen instructions of the Preparation Wizard, providing any data requested. As an example, let's follow the preparation process for digoxin, one of the medications due to be administered to Piya Jordan during this period of care. To begin, click to select **Digoxin**; then click **Prepare**. Now work through the Preparation Wizard sequence as detailed below:

> Amount of medication in the ampule: 2 mL.
> Enter the amount of medication you will draw up into a syringe: <u>**0.5**</u> mL.
> Click **Next**.
> Select the patient you wish to set aside the medication for: **Room 403, Piya Jordan**.
> Click **Finish**.
> Click **Return to Medication Room**.

Copyright © 2007 by Mosby, Inc., an affiliate of Elsevier Inc. All rights reserved.

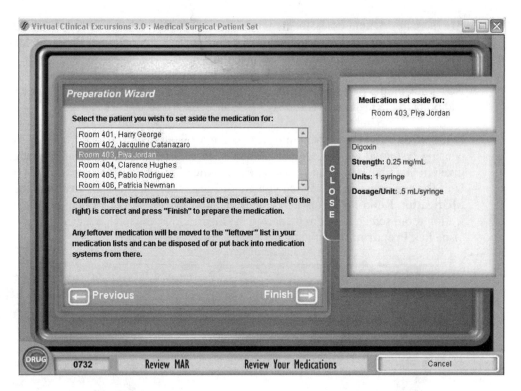

Follow this same basic process for the other medications due to be administered to Piya Jordan during this period of care. (*Hint:* Look in **IV Storage** and **Automated System**.)

PREPARATION WIZARD EXCEPTIONS

- Some medications in *Virtual Clinical Excursions—Medical-Surgical* are preprepared by the pharmacy (e.g., IV antibiotics) and taken to the patient room as a whole. This is common practice in most hospitals.
- Blood products are not administered by students through the *Virtual Clinical Excursions—Medical-Surgical* simulations since blood administration follows specific protocols not covered in this program.
- The *Virtual Clinical Excursions—Medical-Surgical* simulations do not allow for mixing more than one type of medication, such as regular and Lente insulins, in the same syringe. In the clinical setting, when multiple types of insulin are ordered for a patient, the regular insulin is drawn up first, followed by the longer-acting insulin. Insulin is always administered in a special unit-marked syringe.

Now return to Room 403 (click on **403** on the bottom tool bar) to administer Piya Jordan's medications.

At any time during the medication administration process, you can perform a further review of systems, take vital signs, check information contained within the chart, or verify patient identity and allergies. Inside Piya Jordan's room, click **Take Vital Signs**. (*Note:* These findings change over time to reflect the temporal changes you would find in a patient similar to Piya Jordan.)

Copyright © 2007 by Mosby, Inc., an affiliate of Elsevier Inc. All rights reserved.

When you have gathered all the data you need, click on **Patient Care** and then select **Medication Administration**. Any medications you prepared in the previous steps should be listed on the left side of your screen. Let's continue the administration process with the digoxin ordered for Piya Jordan. Click to highlight **Digoxin** in the list of medications. Next, click on the down arrow to the right of **Select** and choose **Administer** from the drop-down menu. This will activate the Administration Wizard. Complete the Wizard sequence as follows:

- Route: **IV**
- Method: **Direct Injection**
- Site: **Peripheral IV**
- Click **Administer to Patient** arrow.
- Would you like to document this administration in the MAR? **Yes**
- Click **Finish** arrow.

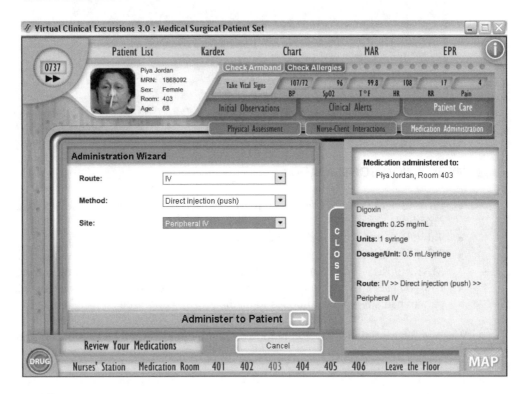

Your selections are recorded by a tracking system and evaluated on a Medication Scorecard stored under Preceptor's Evaluations. This scorecard can be viewed, printed, and given to your instructor. To access the Preceptor's Evaluations, click on **Leave the Floor**. When the Floor Menu appears, click on the icon next to **Look at Your Preceptor's Evaluation**. Then click on **Medication Scorecard** inside the box with Piya Jordan's name (see example on the following page).

Copyright © 2007 by Mosby, Inc., an affiliate of Elsevier Inc. All rights reserved.

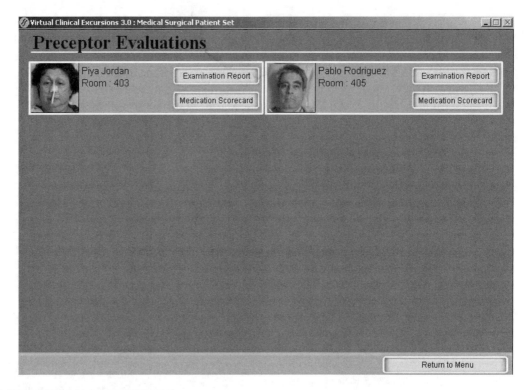

■ MEDICATION SCORECARD

- First, review Table A. Was digoxin given correctly? Did you give the other medications as ordered?
- Table B shows you which (if any) medications you gave incorrectly.
- Table C addresses the resources used for Piya Jordan. Did you access the patient's chart, MAR, EPR, or Kardex as needed to make safe medication administration decisions?
- Did you check the patient's armband to verify her identity? Did you check whether your patient had any known allergies to medications? Were vital signs taken?

When you have finished reviewing the scorecard, click **Return to Evaluations** and then **Return to Menu**.

Copyright © 2007 by Mosby, Inc., an affiliate of Elsevier Inc. All rights reserved.

■ VITAL SIGNS

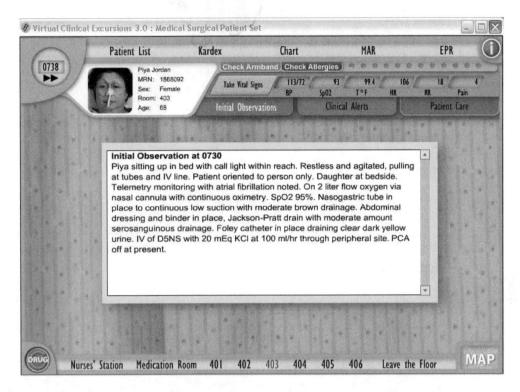

Vital signs, often considered the traditional "signs of life," include body temperature, heart rate, respiratory rate, blood pressure, oxygen saturation of the blood, and pain level.

Inside Piya Jordan's room, click **Take Vital Signs**. (*Note:* If you are following this detailed tour step by step, you will need to **Restart the Program** from the Floor Menu, sign in again, and navigate to Room 403.) Collect vital signs for this patient and record them in the following table. Note the time at which you collected each of these data. (*Remember:* You can take vital signs at any time. The data change over time to reflect the temporal changes you would find in a patient similar to Piya Jordan.)

Vital Signs	Findings/Time
Blood pressure	
O$_2$ saturation	
Heart rate	
Respiratory rate	
Temperature	
Pain rating	

Copyright © 2007 by Mosby, Inc., an affiliate of Elsevier Inc. All rights reserved.

After you are done, click on the **EPR** icon located in the tool bar at the top of the screen. Your username and password are automatically provided. Click on **Login** to enter the EPR. To access Piya Jordan's records, click on the down arrow next to Patient and choose her room number, **403**. Select **Vital Signs** as the category. Next, in the empty time column on the far right, record the vital signs data you just collected in Piya Jordan's room. (*Note:* If you need help with this process, see page 16.) Now compare these findings with the data you collected earlier for this patient's vital signs. Use these earlier findings to establish a baseline for each of the vital signs.

    a.   Are any of the data you collected significantly different from the baseline for a particular vital sign?

        Circle One: Yes   No

    b.   If "Yes," which data are different?

■ PHYSICAL ASSESSMENT

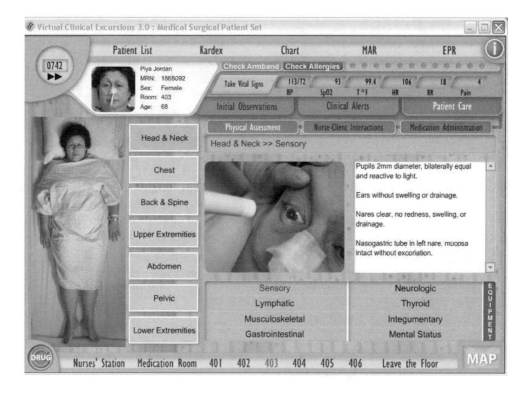

Copyright © 2007 by Mosby, Inc., an affiliate of Elsevier Inc. All rights reserved.

After you have finished examining the EPR for vital signs, click **Exit EPR** to return to Room 403. Click **Patient Care** and then **Physical Assessment**. Think about what information you received in the report at the beginning of this shift, as well as what you may have learned about this patient from the chart. Based on this, what area(s) of examination should you pay most attention to at this time? Is there any equipment you should be monitoring? Conduct a physical assessment of the body areas and systems that you consider priorities for Piya Jordan. For example, select **Head & Neck**; then click on and assess **Sensory** and **Lymphatic**. Complete any other assessment(s) you think are necessary at this time. In the following table, record the data you collected during this examination.

Area of Examination	Findings
Head & Neck Sensory	
Head & Neck Lymphatic	

After you have finished collecting these data, return to the EPR. Compare the data that were already in the record with those you just collected.

a. Are any of the data you collected significantly different from the baselines for this patient?

Circle One: Yes   No

b. If "Yes," which data are different?

Copyright © 2007 by Mosby, Inc., an affiliate of Elsevier Inc. All rights reserved.

■ **NURSE-CLIENT INTERACTIONS**

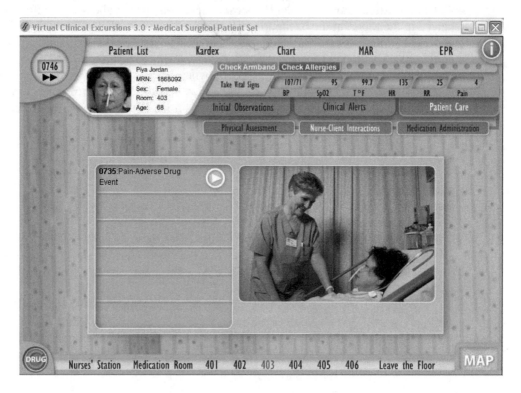

Click on **Patient Care** from inside Piya Jordan's room (403). Now click on **Nurse-Client Interactions** to access a short video titled **Pain—Adverse Drug Event**, which is available for viewing at or after 0735 (based on the virtual clock in the upper left corner of your screen; see *Note* below). To begin the video, click on the arrow next to its title. You will observe a nurse communicating with Piya Jordan and her daughter. There are many variations of nursing practice, some exemplifying "best" practice and some not. Note whether the nurse in this interaction displays professional behavior and compassionate care. Are her words congruent with what is going on with the patient? Does this interaction "feel right" to you? If not, how would you handle this situation differently? Explain.

Note: If the video you wish to view is not listed, this means you have not yet reached the correct virtual time to view that video. Check the virtual clock; you may return to access the video once its designated time has occurred—as long as you do so within the same period of care. Or you can click on the fast-forward icon within the virtual clock to advance the time by 2-minute intervals. You will then need to click again on **Patient Care** and **Nurse-Client Interactions** to refresh the screen.

At least one Nurse-Client Interactions video is available during each period of care. Viewing these videos can help you learn more about what is occurring with a patient at a certain time and also prompt you to discern between nurse communications that are ideal and those that need improvement. Compassionate care and the ability to communicate clearly are essential components of delivering quality nursing care, and it is during your clinical time that you will begin to refine these skills.

Copyright © 2007 by Mosby, Inc., an affiliate of Elsevier Inc. All rights reserved.

■ COLLECTING AND EVALUATING DATA

Each of the activities you perform in the Patient Care environment generates a significant amount of assessment data. Remember that after you collect data, you can record your findings in the EPR. You can also review the EPR, patient's chart, videos, and MAR at any time. You will get plenty of practice collecting and then evaluating data in context of the patient's course.

Now, here's an important question for you:

> Did the previous sequence of exercises provide the most efficient way to assess Piya Jordan?

For example, you went to the patient's room to get vital signs, then back to the EPR to enter data and compare your findings with extant data. Next, you went back to the patient's room to do a physical examination, then again back to the EPR to enter and review data. If this back-and-forth process of data collection and recording seemed inefficient, remember the following:

- Plan all of your nursing activities to maximize efficiency, while at the same time optimizing the quality of patient care. (Think about what data you might need before performing certain tasks. For example, do you need to check a heart rate before administering a cardiac medication or check an IV site before starting an infusion?)

- You collect a tremendous amount of data when you work with a patient. Very few people can accurately remember all these data for more than a few minutes. Develop efficient assessment skills, and record data as soon as possible after collecting them.

- Assessment data are only the starting point for the nursing process.

Make a clear distinction between these first exercises and how you actually provide nursing care. These initial exercises were designed to involve you actively in the use of different software components. This workbook focuses on sensible practices for implementing the nursing process in ways that ensure the highest-quality care of patients.

Most important, remember that a human being changes through time, and that these changes include both the physical and psychosocial facets of a person as a living organism. Think about this for a moment. Some patients may change physically in a very short time (a patient with emerging myocardial infarction) or more slowly (a patient with a chronic illness). Patients' overall physical and psychosocial conditions may improve or deteriorate. They may have effective coping skills and familial support, or they may feel alone and full of despair. In fact, each individual is a complex mix of physical and psychosocial elements, and at least some of these elements usually change through time.

Thus it is crucial that you *DO NOT* think of the nursing process as a simple one-time, five-step procedure consisting of assessment, nursing diagnosis, planning, implementation, and evaluation. Rather, the nursing process should be utilized as a creative and systematic approach to delivering nursing care. Furthermore, because all living organisms are constantly changing, we must apply the nursing process over and over. Each time we follow the nursing process for an individual patient, we refine our understanding of that patient's physical and psychosocial conditions based on collection and analysis of many different types of data. *Virtual Clinical Excursions—Medical-Surgical* will help you develop both the creativity and the systematic approach needed to become a nurse who is equipped to deliver the highest-quality care to all patients.

Copyright © 2007 by Mosby, Inc., an affiliate of Elsevier Inc. All rights reserved.

REDUCING MEDICATION ERRORS

Earlier in this detailed tour, you learned the basic steps of medication preparation and administration. The following simulations will allow you to practice those skills further—with an increased emphasis on reducing medication errors by using the Medication Scorecard to evaluate your work.

Sign in to work at Pacific View Regional Hospital for Period of Care 1. (*Note:* If you are already working with another patient or during another period of care, click on **Leave the Floor** and then **Restart the Program**; then sign in.)

From the Patient List, select Clarence Hughes. Then click on **Go to Nurses' Station**. Complete the following steps to prepare and administer medications to Clarence Hughes.

- Click on **Medication Room**.
- Click on **MAR** and then on tab **404** to determine prn medications that have been ordered for Clarence Hughes to address his constipation and pain. (*Note:* You may click on **Review MAR** at any time to verify the correct medication order. Always remember to check the patient name on the MAR to make sure you have the correct patient's record—you must click on the correct room number tab within the MAR.) Click on **Return to Medication Room** after reviewing the correct MAR.
- Click on **Unit Dosage** (or on the Unit Dosage cabinet); from the close-up view, click on drawer **404**.
- Select the medications you would like to administer. After each selection, click **Put Medication on Tray**. When you are finished selecting medications, click **Close Drawer** and then **View Medication Room**.
- Click on **Automated System** (or on the Automated System unit itself). Click **Login**.
- On the next screen, specify the correct patient and drawer location.
- Select the medication you would like to administer and click on **Put Medication on Tray**. Repeat this process if you wish to administer other medications from the Automated System.
- When you are finished, click **Close Drawer** and **View Medication Room**.
- From the Medication Room, click on **Preparation** (or on the preparation tray).
- From the list of medications on your tray, highlight the correct medication to administer and click **Prepare**.
- This activates the Preparation Wizard. Supply any requested information; then click **Next**.
- Now select the correct patient to receive this medication and click **Finish**.
- Repeat the previous two steps until all medications that you want to administer are prepared.
- You can click on **Review Your Medications** and then on **Return to Medication Room** when ready. Once you are back in the Medication Room, go directly to Clarence Hughes' room by clicking on **404** at bottom of screen.
- Inside the patient's room, administer the medication, utilizing the five rights of medication administration. After you have collected the appropriate assessment data and are ready for administration, click **Patient Care** and then **Medication Administration**. Verify that the correct patient and medication(s) appear in the left-hand window. Highlight the first medication you wish to administer; then click the down arrow next to Select. From the drop-down menu, select **Administer** and complete the Administration Wizard by providing any information requested. When the Wizard stops asking for information, click **Administer to Patient**. Specify **Yes** when asked whether this administration should be recorded in the MAR. Finally, click **Finish**.

Copyright © 2007 by Mosby, Inc., an affiliate of Elsevier Inc. All rights reserved.

■ **SELF-EVALUATION**

Now let's see how you did during your medication administration!

- Click on **Leave the Floor** at the bottom of your screen. From the Floor Menu, select **Look at Your Preceptor's Evaluation**. Then click on **Medication Scorecard** for Clarence Hughes. These resources will help you find out more about each patient's medications and possible sources of medication errors.

1. Start by examining Table A. These are the medications you should have given to Clarence Hughes during this period of care. If each of the medications in Table A has a √ by it, then you made no errors. Congratulations!

If any medication has an X by it, then you made one or more medication errors.

Compare Tables A and B to determine which of the following types of errors you made: Wrong Dose, Wrong Route/Method/Site, or Wrong Time. Follow these steps:
   a. Find medications in Table A that were given incorrectly.
   b. Now see if those same medications are in Table B, which shows what you actually administered to Clarence Hughes.
   c. Comparing Tables A and B, match the Strength, Dose, Route/Method/Site, and Time for each medication you administered incorrectly.
   d. Then, using the form below, list the medications given incorrectly and mark the errors you made for each medication.

Medication	Strength	Dosage	Route	Method	Site	Time
	❑	❑	❑	❑	❑	❑
	❑	❑	❑	❑	❑	❑
	❑	❑	❑	❑	❑	❑
	❑	❑	❑	❑	❑	❑

2. To help you reduce future medication errors, consider the following list of possible reasons for errors.

   - Did not check drug against MAR for correct patient, correct date, correct time, correct drug, and correct dose.
   - Did not check drug dose against MAR three times.
   - Did not open the unit dose package in the patient's room.
   - Did not correctly identify the patient using two identifiers.
   - Did not administer the drug on time.
   - Did not verify patient allergies.
   - Did not check the patient's current condition or vital sign parameters.
   - Did not consider why the patient would be receiving this drug.
   - Did not question why the drug was in the patient's drawer.
   - Did not check the physician's order and/or check with the pharmacist when there was a question about the drug or dose.
   - Did not verify that no adverse effects had occurred from a previous dose.

Copyright © 2007 by Mosby, Inc., an affiliate of Elsevier Inc. All rights reserved.

Based on these possibilities, determine how you made each error and record the reason into the form below:

Medication	Reason for Error

3. Look again at Table B. Are there medications listed that are not in Table A? If so, you gave a medication to Clarence Hughes that he should not have received. Complete the following exercises to help you understand how such an error might have been made.

   a. Perhaps you gave a medication that was on Clarence Hughes' MAR for this period of care, without recognizing that a change had occurred in the patient's condition, which should have caused you to reconsider. Review patient records as necessary and complete the following form:

Medication	Possible Reasons Not to Give This Medication

   b. Another possibility is that you gave Clarence Hughes a medication that should have been given at a different time. Check his MAR and complete the form below to determine whether you made a Wrong Time error:

Medication	Given to Clarence Hughes at What Time	Should Have Been Given at What Time

Copyright © 2007 by Mosby, Inc., an affiliate of Elsevier Inc. All rights reserved.

c. Maybe you gave another patient's medication to Clarence Hughes. In this case, you made a Wrong Patient error. Check the MARs of other patients and use the form below to determine whether you made this type of error:

Medication	Given to Clarence Hughes	Should Have Been Given to

4. The Medication Scorecard provides some other interesting sources of information. For example, if there is a medication selected for Clarence Hughes but it was not given to him, there will be an X by that medication in Table A, but it will not appear in Table B. In that case, you might have given this medication to some other patient, which is another type of Wrong Patient error. To investigate further, look at Table D, which lists the medications you gave to other patients. See whether you can find any medications for Clarence Hughes that were given to another patient by mistake. However, before you make any decisions, be sure to cross-check the MAR for other patients because the same medication may have been ordered for multiple patients. Use the following form to record your findings:

Medication	Should Have Been Given to Clarence Hughes	Given by Mistake to

Copyright © 2007 by Mosby, Inc., an affiliate of Elsevier Inc. All rights reserved.

5. Now take some time to review the medication exercises you just completed. Use the form below to create an overall analysis of what you have learned. Once again, record each of the medication errors you made, including the type of each error. Then, for each error you made, indicate specifically what you would do differently to prevent this type of error from occurring again.

Medication	Type of Error	Error Prevention Tactic

Submit this form to your instructor if required as a graded assignment, or simply use these exercises to improve your understanding of medication errors and how to reduce them.

Name: _____   Date: _____

Copyright © 2007 by Mosby, Inc., an affiliate of Elsevier Inc. All rights reserved.

The following icons are used throughout the workbook to help you quickly identify particular activities and assignments:

 Indicates a reading assignment—tells you which textbook chapter(s) you should read before starting each lesson

 Indicates a writing activity

 Marks the beginning of an interactive CD-ROM activity—signals you to open or return to your *Virtual Clinical Excursions—Medical-Surgical* CD-ROM

 Indicates additional CD-ROM instructions

 Indicates questions and activities that require you to consult your textbook

 Indicates the approximate time required to complete an exercise

Copyright © 2007 by Mosby, Inc., an affiliate of Elsevier Inc. All rights reserved.

LESSON **1**

Culturally Competent Care

 Reading Assignment: Culturally Competent Care (Chapter 3)

Patients: Piya Jordan, Room 403
Clarence Hughes, Room 404
Pablo Rodriguez, Room 405

Goal: Demonstrate understanding and appropriate application of cultural concepts in nursing practice.

Objectives:

1. Define *cultural competence* and associated terminology.
2. Identify appropriate methods of assessing the culture of a patient.
3. Identify specific needs for patients of various cultural and ethnic backgrounds.
4. Describe nursing interventions relevant for patients of various cultures.
5. Correctly utilize the nursing process in providing culturally competent nursing care.

In this lesson you will explore various cultural differences and how nursing care should be adapted to meet each patient's individual needs. Begin this activity by reviewing the general concepts presented in your textbook. Answer the following questions to solidify your understanding of culture.

Exercise 1

 Clinical Preparation: Writing Activity

 20 minutes

1. What aspects of a patient's life and/or environment would be included in a cultural assessment? (See the definition of culture on page 27 in your textbook.)

Copyright © 2007 by Mosby, Inc., an affiliate of Elsevier Inc. All rights reserved.

2. Why is it important for a nurse to assess a patient's culture?

3. Match each of the following terms with its correct definition.

Term	**Definition**
_____ Acculturation	a. Belief that one's own ways are superior to those of others from different cultural, ethnic, or racial backgrounds; can lead to seeing others as different or inferior.
_____ Assimilation	
_____ Cultural competence	b. A gradual process by which an individual or group learns how to take on many, but not all, values, beliefs, and practices of another culture. Often results in increased similarities between the two cultures.
_____ Cultural imposition	
_____ Ethnicity	c. Viewing members of a specific culture, race, or ethnic group as being alike and sharing the same values and beliefs; can lead to false assumptions and affect a patient's care
_____ Ethnocentrism	
_____ Stereotyping	d. Occurs when one's own cultural beliefs and practices are imposed on another person or group of people; can result in disregarding or trivializing a patient's health care beliefs or practices

e. Refers to the manner in which an individual or group from one culture adopts certain features of another culture. Typically a one-way process that may be voluntary or forced onto a group.

f. Refers to groups whose members share a common social and cultural heritage

g. Involves the complex integration of knowledge, attitudes, and skills that enhance cross-cultural communication and foster meaningful, respectful interactions with others.

4. Identify four processes involved in developing cultural competence.

Copyright © 2007 by Mosby, Inc., an affiliate of Elsevier Inc. All rights reserved.

Exercise 2

 CD-ROM Activity

 45 minutes

- Sign in to work at Pacific View Regional Hospital for Period of Care 1. (*Note:* If you are already in the virtual hospital from a previous exercise, click on **Leave the Floor** and then **Restart the Program** to get to the sign-in window.)
- From the Patient List, select Piya Jordan (Room 403), Clarence Hughes (Room 404), and Pablo Rodriguez (Room 405).
- Click on **Go to Nurses' Station**.
- Click on **Chart** and then **403**.
- Click on **History and Physical**.

1. Read Piya Jordans's H&P and document her cultural needs and/or considerations below. Complete the table by repeating the above steps for Clarence Hughes and Pablo Rodriguez.

Patient	Cultural Needs/Considerations
Piya Jordan (Room 403)	
Clarence Hughes (Room 404)	
Pablo Rodriguez (Room 405)	

Copyright © 2007 by Mosby, Inc., an affiliate of Elsevier Inc. All rights reserved.

- Click on **Return to Nurses' Station**.
- Click on **403** to enter Piya Jordan's room.
- Read the Initial Observation.
- Click on **Patient Care** and then **Nurse-Client Interactions**.
- Select and view the video titled **0735: Pain-Adverse Drug Event**. (*Note:* Check the virtual clock to see whether enough time has elapsed. You can use the fast-forward feature to advance the time by 2-minute intervals if the video is not yet available. Then click on **Patient Care** and **Nurse-Client Interactions** to refresh the screen.)

2. Based on this video, what potential cultural factors affecting health and health care (see textbook pages 30-35) should be identified and/or explored when planning care for Piya Jordan? (*Hint:* Use the general areas listed below to guide and organize your answer.)

Medications

Family roles and relationships

Spirituality and Religion

Communication

- Click on **404** at the bottom of the screen to enter Clarence Hughes' room.
- Read the Initial Observation.
- Click on **Patient Care** and then **Nurse-Client Interactions**.
- Select and view the video titled **0730: Assessment/Perception of Care**. (*Note:* Check the virtual clock to see whether enough time has elapsed. You can use the fast-forward feature to advance the time by 2-minute intervals if the video is not yet available. Then click on **Patient Care** and **Nurse-Client Interactions** to refresh the screen.)

Copyright © 2007 by Mosby, Inc., an affiliate of Elsevier Inc. All rights reserved.

3. Based on this video, what potential cultural factors affecting health and health care (see textbook pages 30-35) should be identified and/or explored when planning care for Clarence Hughes? (*Hint:* Use the general areas listed below to guide and organize your answer.)

Spirituality and Religion

Communication

 • Click on **405** at the bottom of the screen to enter Pablo Rodriguez's room.

• Read the Initial Observation.

• Click on **Patient Care** and then **Nurse-Client Interactions**.

• Select and view the video titled **0730: Symptom Management**. (*Note:* Check the virtual clock to see whether enough time has elapsed. You can use the fast-forward feature to advance the time by 2-minute intervals if the video is not yet available. Then click on **Patient Care** and **Nurse-Client Interactions** to refresh the screen.)

4. Describe how Pablo Rodriguez's comments reveal his cultural beliefs.

Copyright © 2007 by Mosby, Inc., an affiliate of Elsevier Inc. All rights reserved.

5. Using the nursing process, develop a culturally sensitive nursing care plan for Pablo Rodriguez in relation to the two patient problems identified in the left column below. Document your plan in the remaining columns.

Patient Problems (Assessment)	Nursing Diagnosis	Goals/Outcomes (Planning)	Nursing Interventions	Evaluation
Pain				
Spiritual/ cultural needs				

Copyright © 2007 by Mosby, Inc., an affiliate of Elsevier Inc. All rights reserved.

Pain

 Reading Assignment: Pain (Chapter 10)

Patients: Clarence Hughes, Room 404
Pablo Rodriguez, Room 405

Goal: Demonstrate understanding and appropriate application of pain management concepts.

Objectives:

1. Define the concept of pain.
2. Describe the six dimensions of pain.
3. Describe the source and type of pain for each patient.
4. Perform a comprehensive pain assessment for each patient.
5. Identify variables that influence each patient's perception of pain.
6. Safely administer analgesic medications to a patient experiencing pain.
7. Plan appropriate nonpharmacologic measures that may be used to treat each patient's pain.

In this lesson you will evaluate the pain experience of two different patients from assessment to management. Clarence Hughes is a 73-year-old male who is status post total knee arthroplasty. Pablo Rodriguez is a 71-year-old male admitted with advanced non-small cell lung carcinoma. Begin this activity by reviewing the general concepts presented in your textbook. Answer the following questions to solidify your understanding of pain.

Exercise 1

 Clinical Preparation: Writing Activity

20 minutes

1. Using the definitions of pain provided in the textbook, describe pain in your own words.

Copyright © 2007 by Mosby, Inc., an affiliate of Elsevier Inc. All rights reserved.

2. Briefly describe the following six dimensions of pain discussed in your textbook.

Physiologic

Sensory

Affective

Behavioral

Cognitive

Sociocultural

Copyright © 2007 by Mosby, Inc., an affiliate of Elsevier Inc. All rights reserved.

3. Define *nociception*.

4. Briefly describe the following four processes of nociception.

Transduction

Transmission

Perception

Modulation

Copyright © 2007 by Mosby, Inc., an affiliate of Elsevier Inc. All rights reserved.

Exercise 2

 CD-ROM Activity

 45 minutes

- Sign in to work at Pacific View Regional Hospital for Period of Care 1. (*Note:* If you are already in the virtual hospital from a previous exercise, click on **Leave the Floor** and then **Restart the Program** to get to the sign-in window.)
- From the Patient List, select Clarence Hughes (Room 404).
- Click on **Get Report**.

1. What information is obtained during report concerning Clarence Hughes' most recent pain assessment?

Now complete your own pain assessment on Clarence Hughes.

- Click on **Go to Nurses' Station**.
- Click on **404** at the bottom of the screen.
- Click on **Take Vital Signs**.

2. How does Clarence Hughes rate his pain at the present time?

- Click on **Patient Care**.

3. Perform a focused assessment on this patient. Document your findings below.

- Click on **Nurse-Client Interactions**.
- Select and view the video titled **0730: Assessment/Perception of Care**. (*Note:* Check the virtual clock to see whether enough time has elapsed. You can use the fast-forward feature to advance the time by 2-minute intervals if the video is not yet available. Then click on **Patient Care** and **Nurse-Client Interactions** to refresh the screen.)

Copyright © 2007 by Mosby, Inc., an affiliate of Elsevier Inc. All rights reserved.

4. How does Clarence Hughes describe his pain? Describe his nonverbal communication. Do his nonverbal cues correlate with his complaint of pain?

5. The nurse asks Clarence Hughes if she may perform an assessment prior to medicating him for pain. Is this appropriate? Why or why not?

→ • Click on **EPR** and then **Login**.
  • From the drop-down menu next to Patient, choose **404**.
  • Select **Vital Signs** as the category. (Use the arrows at the bottom of the screen to move forward and backward in time.)

6. Document Clarence Hughes' pain rating and characteristics over the last 24 hours in the table provided below and on the next page. (*Note:* You will complete the table in question 7.)

→ • Click on **Exit EPR**.
  • Click on **Chart** and then **404** for Clarence Hughes' chart.
  • Within the chart, click on the **Expired MARs** tab.

7. Review the expired MARs for Clarence Hughes noting the times of analgesic administration. Document your findings in the far right column below and on the next page.

Time of Assessment	Pain Rating	Pain Characteristic	Name of Analgesic Administered
Tuesday 0700			
Tuesday 0815			
Tuesday 0930			
Tuesday 1230			
Tuesday 1330			

Copyright © 2007 by Mosby, Inc., an affiliate of Elsevier Inc. All rights reserved.

Time of Assessment	Pain Rating	Pain Characteristic	Name of Analgesic Administered
Tuesday 1500			
Tuesday 1630			
Tuesday 1700			
Tuesday 2030			
Tuesday 2300			
Wednesday 0200			
Wednesday 0715			

- Click on **Return to Room 404**.
- Click on **Kardex**.
- Click on **404** for Clarence Hughes' records.

8. What is the stated outcome related to comfort for Clarence Hughes? Is this a measurable outcome? How might you improve on the writing of the outcome?

9. Based on the stated outcome, review the table you completed in questions 6 and 7. Was the pain medication administered effective? Give a rationale for your answer.

Copyright © 2007 by Mosby, Inc., an affiliate of Elsevier Inc. All rights reserved.

10. Was the patient's pain assessed appropriately following each analgesic administration? Explain your answer.

11. How would you classify Clarence Hughes' pain? Explain your answer. (*Hint:* See pages 130-131 of your textbook.)

12. Is the ordered analgesic medication appropriate for this type of pain? If not, what would you suggest? Are there any nonpharmacologic interventions that might be helpful for Clarence Hughes? Explain your answer.

13. What nursing assessment should be completed prior to administration of oxycodone with acetaminophen?

Copyright © 2007 by Mosby, Inc., an affiliate of Elsevier Inc. All rights reserved.

14. For what common side effects should the nurse monitor Clarence Hughes related to opioid use?

- Click on **Return to Room 404**.
- Click on **Chart.**
- Click on **404** for Clarence Hughes' chart.
- Click on the **Nurse's Notes** tab and review the notes.

15. According to the note for Wednesday at 0715, which of the side effects (identified in question 14) is Clarence Hughes experiencing? What should the nurse do to treat and/or prevent this side effect?

Since Clarence Hughes received his last dose of pain medication at 0200, it is now appropriate to administer another dose. Prepare to administer a dose of analgesic to him by completing the following steps:

- Click on **Return to Nurses' Station**.
- Click **Medication Room** on the bottom of your screen.
- Access the **Automated System** by either selecting that icon at the top of screen or by clicking on the Automated System cart in the center of the screen.
- Click on **Login**.
- Choose Clarence Hughes in box 1 and Automated System Drawer (G-O) in box 2. Click **Open Drawer** and review the list of available medications. (*Note:* You may click **Review MAR** at any time to verify the medication order. Remember to look at the patient name on the MAR to make sure you have the correct record—you must click on the correct room number within the MAR. Click on **Return to Medication Room** after reviewing the correct MAR.)
- From the Open Drawer view, select the correct medication to administer. Click **Put Medication on Tray** and then **Close Drawer**.
- Click on **View Medication Room**.
- Begin the preparation process by clicking on **Preparation** at the top of the screen or by clicking on the tray on the counter on the left side of the Medication Room.
- Click **Prepare**, fill in any requested data in the Preparation Wizard, and click **Next**. Then select the correct patient and click **Finish**.
- You can click on **Review Your Medications** and then on **Return to Medication Room** when ready. Once you are back in the Medication Room, you may go directly to Clarence Hughes' room to administer this medication by clicking on **404** at the bottom of the screen.

Copyright © 2007 by Mosby, Inc., an affiliate of Elsevier Inc. All rights reserved.

- Administer the medication, utilizing the five rights of medication administration. After you have collected the appropriate assessment data and are ready for administration, click **Patient Care** and then **Medication Administration**. Verify that the correct patient and medication(s) appear in the left-hand window. Then click the down arrow next to Select. From the drop-down menu, select **Administer** and complete the Administration Wizard by providing any information requested. When the Wizard stops asking for information, click **Administer to Patient**. Specify **Yes** when asked whether this administration should be recorded in the MAR. Finally, click **Finish**.

Now let's see how you did!

 - Click on **Leave the Floor** at the bottom of your screen. From the Floor Menu, select **Look at Your Preceptor's Evaluation**. Then click on **Medication Scorecard**.

16. Disregard the report for the routine scheduled medications but note below whether or not you correctly administered the analgesic medication. If not, why do you think you were incorrect in administering this drug? According to Table C in this scorecard, what are the appropriate resources that should be used prior to administering this medication? Did you utilize them correctly?

Exercise 3

 CD-ROM Activity

 45 minutes

- Sign in to work at Pacific View Regional Hospital for Period of Care 1. (*Note:* If you are already in the virtual hospital from a previous exercise, click on **Leave the Floor** and then **Restart the Program** to get to the sign-in window.)
- From the Patient List, select Pablo Rodriguez (Room 405).
- Click on **Get Report**.

1. What information is obtained during report concerning Pablo Rodriguez's most recent pain assessment?

Now complete your own pain assessment on this patient.

 - Click on **Go to Nurses' Station**.
- Click on **405**.
- Click on **Take Vital Signs**.

Copyright © 2007 by Mosby, Inc., an affiliate of Elsevier Inc. All rights reserved.

2. How does Pablo Rodriguez rate his pain at the present time?

→ • Click on **Patient Care**.

3. Perform a focused assessment on this patient. Document your findings below.

→ • Click on **Chart**.
   • Click on **405** for the correct patient chart.
   • Click on **Nursing Admission**.

4. Scroll down to page 22 of the Nursing Admission form. What are the aggravating and alleviating factors related to Pablo Rodriguez's pain?

5. What cultural influences are affecting this patient's perception and management of pain?

→ • Click on **Return to Room 405**.
   • Click on **Patient Care** and then **Nurse-Client Interactions**.
   • Select and view the video titled **0730: Symptom Management**. (*Note:* Check the virtual clock to see whether enough time has elapsed. You can use the fast-forward feature to advance the time by 2-minute intervals if the video is not yet available. Then click on **Patient Care** and **Nurse-Client Interactions** to refresh the screen.)

Copyright © 2007 by Mosby, Inc., an affiliate of Elsevier Inc. All rights reserved.

→ • Click on **EPR** and then **Login**.
  • Select **405** as the patient and **Vital Signs** as the category.

6. In the table below, document Pablo Rodriguez's pain ratings and characteristics since admission. (*Note:* You will complete the table in question 7.)

Time of Assessment	Pain Rating	Pain Characteristic	Time of Medication Administration	Name of Analgesic Administered
Tuesday 2300				
Wednesday 0300				
Wednesday 0700				

→ • Click on **Exit EPR**.
  • Click on **Chart**.
  • Select **405**.
  • Click on **Expired MARs**.

7. Review the expired MAR, noting the times of analgesic administration. Document your findings in the table above.

→ • Click on **Return to Room 405**.
  • Click on **Kardex**.
  • Click on **405** for the correct records.

8. What is the stated outcome related to comfort for Pablo Rodriguez? Is this a measurable outcome? How might you improve on the writing of the outcome?

Copyright © 2007 by Mosby, Inc., an affiliate of Elsevier Inc. All rights reserved.

9. Based on the stated outcome, review the table you completed in questions 6 and 7, as well as your pain assessment in question 2. Was the pain medication administered effective? Give a rationale for your answer.

10. Was the patient's pain assessed appropriately following each analgesic administration? Explain your answer.

11. How would you classify Pablo Rodriguez's pain? Explain your answer. (*Hint:* See pages 130-131 of your textbook.)

12. Is the ordered analgesic medication appropriate for this type of pain? If not, what would you suggest? Are there any nonpharmacologic interventions that might be helpful for this patient? Explain your answer.

Copyright © 2007 by Mosby, Inc., an affiliate of Elsevier Inc. All rights reserved.

➤ • Click on **Return to Room 405**.
  • Click on **Patient Care** and then **Nurse-Client Interactions**.
  • Select and view the video titled **0735: Patient Perceptions**. (*Note:* Check the virtual clock to see whether enough time has elapsed. You can use the fast-forward feature to advance the time by 2-minute intervals if the video is not yet available. Then click on **Patient Care** and **Nurse-Client Interactions** to refresh the screen.)

13. Discuss the nurse's evaluation of Pablo Rodriguez's understanding and use of the PCA pump. Do you think the nurse's actions are therapeutic? If not, what other approaches would you suggest?

14. What nursing assessments and interventions are appropriate for patients receiving IV morphine sulfate? (*Hint:* For help, click on the **Drug** icon in the lower left corner of the screen.)

Copyright © 2007 by Mosby, Inc., an affiliate of Elsevier Inc. All rights reserved.

End-of-Life and Palliative Care

 Reading Assignment: End-of-Life and Palliative Care (Chapter 11)

Patient: Pablo Rodriguez, Room 405

Goal: Demonstrate understanding and appropriate application of end-of-life concepts in nursing practice.

Objectives:

1. Identify appropriate application of palliative care concepts for a patient with a terminal illness.
2. Assess for and identify common clinical manifestations present at end of life.
3. Choose interventions appropriate to relieve clinical manifestations in a terminally ill patient.
4. Describe appropriate communication techniques when dealing with a terminally ill patient and family.
5. Discuss ethical issues related to providing pain relief during end-of-life care.

In this lesson you will describe, plan, and evaluate the care of a patient with a terminal illness that is no longer responding to therapy. Pablo Rodriguez is a 71-year-old male suffering from advanced non-small cell lung carcinoma diagnosed 1 year ago.

Exercise 1

 Clinical Preparation: Writing Activity

15 minutes

1. What are the goals for end-of-life care?

Copyright © 2007 by Mosby, Inc., an affiliate of Elsevier Inc. All rights reserved.

2. Describe the diagnostic criteria for clinical diagnosis of brain death in adults as recommended by the Quality Standards Subcommittee of the American Academy of Neurology in 1995.

3. What is palliative care? Describe its purpose and identify the six necessary skill sets used during the provision of palliative care.

4. What two criteria must be present for admission to a hospice program?

Exercise 2

 CD-ROM Activity

 45 minutes

- Sign in to work at Pacific View Regional Hospital for Period of Care 3. (*Note:* If you are already in the virtual hospital from a previous exercise, click on **Leave the Floor** and then **Restart the Program** to get to the sign-in window.)
- From the Patient List, select Pablo Rodriguez (Room 405).
- Click on **Go to Nurses' Station**.
- Click on **Chart** and then **405**.
- Click on the **Emergency Department** tab and review the record.

1. Why was Pablo Rodriguez admitted to the hospital?

Copyright © 2007 by Mosby, Inc., an affiliate of Elsevier Inc. All rights reserved.

2. What are his primary and secondary diagnoses?

→ • Click on **Nursing Admission**.

3. What does the admitting nurse document as this patient's anticipated needs for support at the time of discharge?

4. Does the patient have a signed advance directive?

5. What does the Omnibus Reconciliation Act of 1990 (Patient Self-Determination Act) require health care agencies to provide to patients without an advance directive? (*Hint:* See textbook page 155.)

→ • Click on **Nurse's Notes**.

6. Based on available documentation, do you think the admitting nurse complied with the Omnibus Reconciliation Act of 1990?

→ • Click on **Kardex**.
• Click on tab **405**.

Copyright © 2007 by Mosby, Inc., an affiliate of Elsevier Inc. All rights reserved.

7. What is Pablo Rodriguez's code status? Is this appropriate based on the reason for his admission? Explain. (*Hint:* See your answer for question 1.)

8. According to the textbook, what is the new term replacimg a DNR (do not resuscitate) order? Describe what this term means.

 • Click on **Return to Nurses' Station**.
   • Click on **405**.
   • Select **Patient Care** and then **Nurse-Client Interactions**.
   • Select and view the video titled **1530: Decision—End-of-Life Care**. (*Note:* Check the virtual clock to see whether enough time has elapsed. You can use the fast-forward feature to advance the time by 2-minute intervals if the video is not yet available. Then click on **Patient Care** and **Nurse-Client Interactions** to refresh the screen.)

9. What is Pablo Rodriguez telling the nurse in this interaction?

10. What therapeutic communication techniques is the nurse using? Are they effective? What other technique(s) might have been used?

Copyright © 2007 by Mosby, Inc., an affiliate of Elsevier Inc. All rights reserved.

11. What would you do if Pablo Rodriguez asked you to administer a lethal dose of morphine to "stop my pain and help me die with dignity"?

12. What legal term would apply if you were to comply with this request?

Exercise 3

 CD-ROM Activity

 45 minutes

- Sign in to work at Pacific View Regional Hospital for Period of Care 1. (*Note:* If you are already in the virtual hospital from a previous exercise, click on **Leave the Floor** and then **Restart the Program** to get to the sign-in window.)
- From the Patient List, select Pablo Rodriguez (Room 405).
- Click on **Go to Nurses' Station**.
- Click on **405**.

1. According to the Initial Observation report on Pablo Rodriguez, what physical symptom of distress is he displaying?

Copyright © 2007 by Mosby, Inc., an affiliate of Elsevier Inc. All rights reserved.

2. How would you intervene to alleviate his symptoms? Provide rationales for your interventions. (*Hint:* If you need help, go to the patient's chart to review the physician's orders. The Drug Guide in the Nurses' Station may provide rationales for medication administration.)

 • Click on **Nurses' Station**.
   • Click on **EPR**.
   • Click **Login**.
   • Select **405** as the patient and **Vital Signs** as the category.
   • Find the vital sign assessment documented at 0700. (*Hint:* Use the backward and forward arrows to scroll between times.)

3. Describe Pablo Rodriguez's pain assessment.

4. What interventions would be appropriate to relieve this pain?

Copyright © 2007 by Mosby, Inc., an affiliate of Elsevier Inc. All rights reserved.

Now let's check the patient's current vital signs.

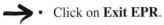 • Click on **Exit EPR**.
• Click on **405** at the bottom of your screen.
• Click on **Take Vital Signs**. (*Note:* Pain assessment is considered the fifth vital sign.)

5. Based on the EPR data and Pablo Rodriguez's current pain rating, is the morphine providing effective relief? Explain.

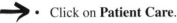 • Click on **Patient Care**.
• From the list of body areas, click on **Abdomen**.
• From the system subcategories, click on **Gastrointestinal**.

6. Document your assessment findings below. What is the significance of these findings? How do they relate to Pablo Rodriguez's diagnosis and/or treatment?

7. How would you intervene to prevent potential complications related to the above findings?

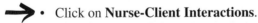 • Click on **Nurse-Client Interactions**.
• Select and view the video titled **0730: Symptom Management**. (*Note:* Check the virtual clock to see whether enough time has elapsed. You can use the fast-forward feature to advance the time by 2-minute intervals if the video is not yet available. Then click on **Patient Care** and **Nurse-Client Interactions** to refresh the screen.)

8. Describe Pablo Rodriguez's emotional distress as displayed in this video.

Copyright © 2007 by Mosby, Inc., an affiliate of Elsevier Inc. All rights reserved.

9. What nursing interventions would be appropriate to help this patient cope?

➤ • Now select and view the video titled **0735: Patient Perceptions**. (*Note:* Check the virtual clock to see whether enough time has elapsed. You can use the fast-forward feature to advance the time by 2-minute intervals if the video is not yet available. Then click on **Patient Care** and **Nurse-Client Interactions** to refresh the screen.)

10. Now that his pain has been controlled, what two physical symptoms does Pablo Rodriguez complain of? How would you intervene to relieve these discomforts?

11. Recall the goals for end-of-life care as noted in your preclinical assignment. Are these being met for Pablo Rodriguez? Explain.

Copyright © 2007 by Mosby, Inc., an affiliate of Elsevier Inc. All rights reserved.

Addictive Behaviors

 Reading Assignment: Addictive Behaviors (Chapter 12)

Patient: Harry George, Room 401

Goal: Demonstrate understanding and appropriate application of health care concepts related to addiction and substance abuse.

Objectives:

1. Identify factors contributing to a patient's addiction.
2. Describe assessment findings related to the use of nicotine and alcohol.
3. Describe assessment findings related to withdrawal from nicotine and alcohol.
4. Examine alcohol withdrawal protocols for the care of a patient admitted to an acute care setting.
5. Identify appropriate nursing interventions when caring for a patient with substance abuse.

In this lesson you will learn about the care of a patient undergoing specific substance abuse issues. Harry George is a 54-year-old male admitted with infection and swelling of his left foot and a history of type 2 diabetes. Begin this activity by reviewing the general concepts presented in your textbook. Answer the following questions to solidify your understanding of substance abuse.

Exercise 1

Clinical Preparation: Writing Activity

10 minutes

1. Define *substance abuse*.

Copyright © 2007 by Mosby, Inc., an affiliate of Elsevier Inc. All rights reserved.

2. Define *addiction*.

3. Describe the neurophysiology of addiction.

Exercise 2

 CD-ROM Activity

 30 minutes

- Sign in to work at Pacific View Regional Hospital for Period of Care 1. (*Note:* If you are already in the virtual hospital from a previous exercise, click on **Leave the Floor** and then **Restart the Program** to get to the sign-in window.)
- From the Patient List, select Harry George (Room 401).
- Click on **Go to Nurses' Station**.
- Click on **Chart** and then **401** to view Harry George's chart.
- Click on the **Emergency Department** tab and review this record.

1. What are Harry George's primary and secondary diagnoses?

Copyright © 2007 by Mosby, Inc., an affiliate of Elsevier Inc. All rights reserved.

2. What specific contributing factor(s) to addiction is (are) noted in the Emergency Department record? (*Hint:* Read the admitting physician notes.) Describe how the factor(s) contribute(s) to alcohol abuse.

3. Although unknown for this patient, what other potential contributing factors to addiction might have led to Harry George's substance abuse? (*Hint:* See pages 166-167 of your textbook.)

4. When did Harry George begin drinking excessively? Was there a precipitating event that contributed to this problem? If so, explain.

5. What other documentation is found in the Emergency Department record to support the diagnosis of alcohol abuse?

6. Is there any evidence of nicotine addiction?

Copyright © 2007 by Mosby, Inc., an affiliate of Elsevier Inc. All rights reserved.

➡ • Still within the chart, click on the **History and Physical** tab.

7. Read the physical examination report on page 4 of the H&P. What assessment findings may be related to Harry George's alcohol abuse?

8. What further history can you find regarding nicotine abuse?

9. What physical examination finding may be related to cigarette smoking?

➡ • Click on **Laboratory Reports**.

10. What is Harry George's blood alcohol level?

11. What clinical manifestations would you expect to find based on this level? (*Hint:* See page 177 of your textbook.)

➡ • Click on **Return to Nurses' Station**.
 • Click on **401** to go to Harry George's room.
 • Click on **Patient Care** and then **Nurse-Client Interactions**.
 • Select and view the video titled **0735: Symptom Management**. (*Note:* Check the virtual clock to see whether enough time has elapsed. You can use the fast-forward feature to advance the time by 2-minute intervals if the video is not yet available. Then click on **Patient Care** and **Nurse-Client Interactions** to refresh the screen.)

Copyright © 2007 by Mosby, Inc., an affiliate of Elsevier Inc. All rights reserved.

12. What visual assessment findings noted in this video interaction might suggest withdrawal symptoms for Harry George?

Exercise 3

 CD-ROM Activity

 45 minutes

- Sign in to work at Pacific View Regional Hospital for Period of Care 4. (*Note:* If you are already in the virtual hospital from a previous exercise, click on **Leave the Floor** and then **Restart the Program** to get to the sign-in window.)
- Click on **Chart** and then **401** to view Harry George's chart. (*Remember:* You are not able to visit patients or administer medications during Period of Care 4. You are able to review patients' records only.)
- Click on and review the **Mental Health** tab.

1. Read the Psychiatric/Mental Health Assessment for Harry George. What contributing factors to addiction are noted in this assessment?

 - Click on **History and Physical**.

2. What effects of chronic alcohol abuse are present in Harry George? (*Hint:* See page 177 in your textbook.)

Copyright © 2007 by Mosby, Inc., an affiliate of Elsevier Inc. All rights reserved.

3. If Harry George's alcohol abuse history was 20 years instead of just 4 years, what additional effects might occur? Identify at least one effect for each of the body systems listed below.

Central Nervous System

Peripheral Nervous System

Hematologic System

Musculoskeletal System

Cardiovascular System

Hepatic System

Gastrointestinal System

Urinary System

Integumentary System

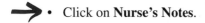 • Click on **Nurse's Notes**.

4. How does the nurse describe Harry George's behavior now?

Copyright © 2007 by Mosby, Inc., an affiliate of Elsevier Inc. All rights reserved.

5. The textbook identifies the following symptoms of patients experiencing alcohol withdrawal. Put an X next to each symptom that applies to Harry George.

_____ a. Tremors

_____ b. Anxiety

_____ c. Increased heart rate

_____ d. Increased blood pressure

_____ e. Nausea

_____ f. Sweating

_____ g. Hyperreflexia

_____ h. Insomnia

_____ i. Disorientation

_____ j. Hallucinations

_____ k. Increased hyperactivity without seizures

_____ l. Seizures

_____ m. Alcohol withdrawal delirium

6. Symptoms of withdrawal can be categorized as minor or major. How would you classify Harry George's symptoms? (*Hint:* See page 178 in your textbook.)

• Click on **Emergency Department**.

7. At what time did Harry George have his last alcoholic drink? Calculate the number of hours that have passed since his last drink and relate this to the usual time frame noted for withdrawal symptoms.

• Click on **History and Physical**.

8. At the end of the History and Physical, the physician writes a plan of care. What pharmacologic interventions is the physician planning to prevent and/or treat alcohol withdrawal?

Copyright © 2007 by Mosby, Inc., an affiliate of Elsevier Inc. All rights reserved.

9. What is the intended benefit of thiamine administration for this patient? (*Hint:* Refer to pages 177-178 in your textbook.)

10. What is the classification of chlordiazepoxide? Identify this drug's most common brand name. What is the intended therapeutic effect of this drug for Harry George? (*Hint:* For help, consult the Drug Guide located in the Nurses' Station.)

➤ • Still in the chart, click on **Nurse's Notes**.

11. Read the notes dated Wednesday at 1245 and at 1315. Is the chlordiazepoxide effective? Give a rationale for your answer.

12. What is the classification of lorazepam? Identify its most common brand name. What is the intended therapeutic effect of this drug for Harry George?

13. Are there any potential drug interactions between chlordiazepoxide and lorazepam? If so, please describe.

NO they both aim to produce the same therapeutic effects could depress CNS

Copyright © 2007 by Mosby, Inc., an affiliate of Elsevier Inc. All rights reserved.

14. Since both Librium and Ativan are ordered for a similar therapeutic effect, what factors would influence the nurse's decision regarding which of these medications to use. (*Hint:* Consult the MAR.)

The nurse would have to decide. If the patient has mild, moderate or severe agitation. Lorazepam is for severe and librium is for mild-moderate

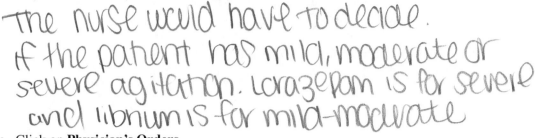

• Click on **Physician's Orders**.

15. What is the most recent physician order?

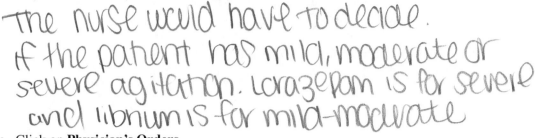

• Click on **Physician's Notes**.

16. Read the most recent physician's progress note. What is the rationale for writing the order you identified in question 15?

17. Based on your readings in the textbook (see pages 183-184), what interventions would you expect to be part of an Alcohol Withdrawal Protocol?

Copyright © 2007 by Mosby, Inc., an affiliate of Elsevier Inc. All rights reserved.

→ • Once again, click on **Nurse's Notes**.

18. Read the note for Wednesday at 1800. What clinical manifestations of nicotine withdrawal is the patient exhibiting?

19. According to your textbook, after how many hours of abstinence do nicotine withdrawal symptoms begin to appear? When do they peak? How long do they last?

20. How long has Harry George been without cigarettes? (*Hint:* Look at time and date of first nurse's note.)

21. What is the effect of simultaneous alcohol and nicotine withdrawal?

22. What typical manifestations of nicotine withdrawal might be found in another patient withdrawing *only* from nicotine?

Copyright © 2007 by Mosby, Inc., an affiliate of Elsevier Inc. All rights reserved.

23. To plan nursing care for Harry George, identify three priority nursing diagnoses for the patient problems identified in the table below. For each diagnosis, identify related patient outcomes and appropriate nursing interventions to achieve these outcomes.

Patient Problems (Assessment)	Nursing Diagnosis	Goals/Outcomes (Planning)	Nursing Interventions
Tremors			
Anxiety			
Malnutrition			

Copyright © 2007 by Mosby, Inc., an affiliate of Elsevier Inc. All rights reserved.

LESSON 5

Cancer

⟨∞⟩ **Reading Assignment:** Cancer (Chapter 16)
Nursing Management: Lower Respiratory Problems
(Chapter 28, pages 578-584)
Nursing Management: Hematologic Problems (Chapter 31,
pages 701-707, 723-726, and 732-734)

Patient: Pablo Rodriguez, Room 405

Goal: Utilize the nursing process to competently care for patients with cancer.

Objectives:

1. Describe clinical manifestations and treatment for a patient with cancer.
2. Recognize special needs of patients undergoing treatment for cancer.
3. Appropriately treat a patient's symptoms related to disease process and/or side effects of treatment.
4. Discuss medications prescribed for a patient, including both expected therapeutic effects and adverse/side effects.
5. Plan appropriate general interventions to prevent and/or treat complications related to chemotherapy.

In this lesson you will learn the essentials of caring for a patient diagnosed with cancer. You will collect data, assess, plan, implement, and evaluate care given. Pablo Rodriguez is a 71-year-old male admitted with advanced non-small cell lung carcinoma. Begin this lesson by reviewing the general concepts of cancer as presented in your textbook.

Copyright © 2007 by Mosby, Inc., an affiliate of Elsevier Inc. All rights reserved.

Exercise 1

Clinical Preparation: Writing Activity

20 minutes

1. Define the following terms.

   a. Carcinogen

   b. Oncogene

   c. Nadir

2. Briefly describe the stages of cancer development noted below and on the next page.

   a. Initiation

   b. Promotion

Copyright © 2007 by Mosby, Inc., an affiliate of Elsevier Inc. All rights reserved.

    c. Progression

3. Briefly define and describe the latent period.

4. What are the three types of therapies used to treat cancer? Describe their respective mechanisms of action.

5. What are some common side effects associated with radiation and chemotherapy?

Copyright © 2007 by Mosby, Inc., an affiliate of Elsevier Inc. All rights reserved.

6. Identify the common sites of distant metastasis for lung cancer.

7. List the clinical manifestations associated with lung cancer.

Exercise 2

 CD-ROM Activity

 35 minutes

- Sign in to work at Pacific View Regional Hospital for Period of Care 1. (*Note:* If you are already in the virtual hospital from a previous exercise, click on **Leave the Floor** and then **Restart the Program** to get to the sign-in window.)
- From the Patient List, select Pablo Rodriguez (Room 405).
- Click on **Go to Nurses' Station**.
- Click on **Chart** and then **405**.
- Click on **History and Physical**.

1. What is Pablo Rodriguez's primary diagnosis?

2. How long ago was he diagnosed?

3. What risk factor for lung cancer is documented on the H&P?

Copyright © 2007 by Mosby, Inc., an affiliate of Elsevier Inc. All rights reserved.

4. What are other risk factors for lung cancer? (*Hint:* See pages 578-579 of your textbook.)

5. What clinical manifestations documented in the physician's review of systems are related to this disease process?

6. What treatment has Pablo Rodriguez received so far?

7. How long ago did he receive his last chemotherapy?

8. What are the mechanism of action and the major side effects of docetaxel?

9. What is the nadir of docetaxel? Would the patient still be having side effects from this drug? Why or why not?

Copyright © 2007 by Mosby, Inc., an affiliate of Elsevier Inc. All rights reserved.

10. What specific assessments related to potential bone marrow suppression should the nurse monitor? What interventions would be appropriate to prevent complications of bone marrow suppression? (*Hint:* See assigned readings in Chapter 31 of your textbook.)

 • Click on **Emergency Deaprtment** in the chart.

11. Scroll down to the ED physician's Progress Notes for Tuesday 1800. What type of cancer was noted on the bronchoscopy performed one year ago? Is this the same as or different from non-small cell cancer noted in the H&P?

Exercise 3

 CD-ROM Activity

 30 minutes

• Sign in to work at Pacific View Regional Hospital for Period of Care 1. (*Note:* If you are already in the virtual hospital from a previous exercise, click on **Leave the Floor** and then **Restart the Program** to get to the sign-in window.)
• From the Patient List, select Pablo Rodriguez (Room 405).
• Click on **Get Report** and read the change-of-shift report.

1. What unresolved problem is noted in the report?

Copyright © 2007 by Mosby, Inc., an affiliate of Elsevier Inc. All rights reserved.

→ • Click on **Go to Nurses' Station**.
  • Click on **Chart** and then **405**.
  • Click on **Nurse's Notes**.

2. Look at the note for Wednesday at 0415. How did the nurse respond to Pablo Rodriguez's complaints? Were the nurse's actions appropriate?

3. How might you have responded differently?

→ • Click on **Return to Nurses' Station**.
  • Go to the patient's room by clicking on **405**.
  • Click on **Patient Care** and then **Nurse-Client Interactions**.
  • Select and view the video titled **0735: Patient Perceptions**. (*Note:* Check the virtual clock to see whether enough time has elapsed. You can use the fast-forward feature to advance the time by 2-minute intervals if the video is not yet available. Then click on **Patient Care** and **Nurse-Client Interactions** to refresh the screen.)

4. What are Pablo Rodriguez's two major concerns at this point?

5. What other assessment should you do before treating the patient's complaint of nausea?

→ • Click on **MAR**; then select **405** to access Pablo Rodriguez's record.

6. What medications are ordered to manage the patient's nausea?

Copyright © 2007 by Mosby, Inc., an affiliate of Elsevier Inc. All rights reserved.

7. What might the nurse question regarding these medication orders?

→ • Click on **Return to Room 405**.
  • Click on **Chart** and then **405**.
  • Click on **Nursing Admission**.

8. What is the patient's weight? What is this in kilograms?

→ • Click on **Return to Room 405**.
  • Click on the **Drug** icon in the lower left corner of the screen.

9. Calculate the maximum 24-hour dose for patients receiving this drug for nausea related to chemotherapy.

10. Calculate the maximum 24-hour dose of this drug for management of postoperative nausea and vomiting.

11. Calculate the maximum amount of this medication Pablo Rodriguez could receive per 24 hours as ordered. Is it within the dosage guidelines? Is there any reason to be concerned about this dosage schedule over long periods of time?

Copyright © 2007 by Mosby, Inc., an affiliate of Elsevier Inc. All rights reserved.

12. What are the possible ramifications of giving high doses of this drug?

13. What are the ramifications of *not* giving this medication for the patient's nausea? ·

14. If the nurse administers the prn Reglan at 0730, what should be done with the regularly scheduled 0800 dose?

Exercise 4

  CD-ROM Activity

40 minutes

- Sign in to work at Pacific View Regional Hospital for Period of Care 2. (*Note:* If you are already in the virtual hospital from a previous exercise, click on **Leave the Floor** and then **Restart the Program** to get to the sign-in window.)
- From the Patient List, select Pablo Rodriguez (Room 405).
- Click on **Go to Nurses' Station**.
- Click on **Chart** and then **405**.
- Click on **Laboratory Reports**.

1. Below, record Pablo Rodriguez's alkaline phosphatase and calcium levels obtained on Tuesday at 2000.

2. How do these abnormal results relate to the patient's diagnosis of cancer? (*Hint:* You may need to refer to a laboratory diagnostic guide.)

Copyright © 2007 by Mosby, Inc., an affiliate of Elsevier Inc. All rights reserved.

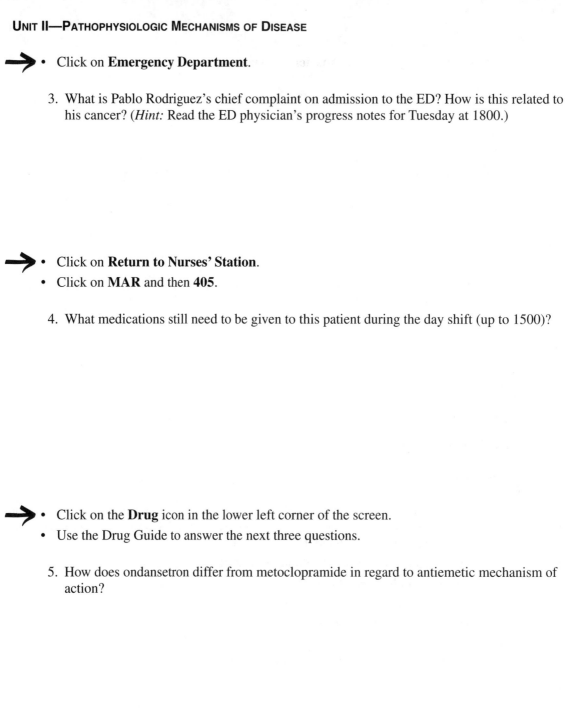

→ • Click on **Emergency Department**.

3. What is Pablo Rodriguez's chief complaint on admission to the ED? How is this related to his cancer? (*Hint:* Read the ED physician's progress notes for Tuesday at 1800.)

→ • Click on **Return to Nurses' Station**.
 • Click on **MAR** and then **405**.

4. What medications still need to be given to this patient during the day shift (up to 1500)?

→ • Click on the **Drug** icon in the lower left corner of the screen.
 • Use the Drug Guide to answer the next three questions.

5. How does ondansetron differ from metoclopramide in regard to antiemetic mechanism of action?

6. How fast would you infuse the IV ondansetron?

7. What is the expected benefit that Pablo Rodriguez will receive from dexamethasone? Over what time period should it be administered?

Copyright © 2007 by Mosby, Inc., an affiliate of Elsevier Inc. All rights reserved.

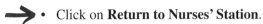 • Click on **Return to Nurses' Station**.
  • Click on **Chart** and then **405**.
  • Click on **Patient Education**.

8. Has any teaching yet been completed? In your opinion, what is a priority and thus should have been completed on admission?

 • Click on **Return to Nurses' Station**.
  • Go to Pablo Rodriguez's room by clicking on **405**.
  • Click on **Patient Care** and then **Nurse-Client Interactions**.
  • Select and view the video titled **1150: Assessment—Pain**. (*Note:* Check the virtual clock to see whether enough time has elapsed. You can use the fast-forward feature to advance the time by 2-minute intervals if the video is not yet available. Then click on **Patient Care** and **Nurse-Client Interactions** to refresh the screen.)

9. Why is the patient not eating?

10. Is this a normal side effect of chemotherapy?

11. How would you treat this?

Copyright © 2007 by Mosby, Inc., an affiliate of Elsevier Inc. All rights reserved.

→ • Click on **Kardex** and read the outcomes.

12. What additional outcome(s) might you include for this patient?

13. What is the patient's code status? How do you feel about this in relation to the patient's diagnosis and condition? What is the nurse's professional responsibility related to the patient's code status?

Copyright © 2007 by Mosby, Inc., an affiliate of Elsevier Inc. All rights reserved.

Fluid Imbalance

 Reading Assignment: Fluid, Electrolyte, and Acid-Base Imbalances (Chapter 17)

Patients: Piya Jordan, Room 403
Patricia Newman, Room 406

Goal: Utilize the nursing process to competently care for patients with fluid imbalances.

Objectives:

1. Identify normal physiologic influences on fluid and electrolyte balance.
2. Compare and contrast causes and clinical manifestations related to extracellular fluid (ECF) volume deficit and ECF volume excess.
3. Utilize laboratory data and clinical manifestations to assess fluid balance and imbalance.
4. Describe collaborative management strategies used to maintain and/or restore fluid balance.
5. Critically analyze differences in fluid balance assessment findings of two patients.
6. Develop an appropriate plan of care for patients displaying ECF volume imbalances.

In this lesson you will assess, plan, and implement care for two patients with similar but differing extracellular fluid volume imbalances. Piya Jordan is a 68-year-old female admitted with nausea and vomiting for several days following weeks of poor appetite and increasing weakness. Patricia Newman is a 61-year-old female admitted with dyspnea at rest, cough, and fever. Begin this activity by reviewing the general concepts of fluid homeostasis as presented in your textbook. Answer the following questions to cement your understanding of the normal physiologic concepts related to fluid balance.

Exercise 1

Clinical Preparation: Writing Activity

⏱ 30 minutes

1. Describe the functions of body water.

Copyright © 2007 by Mosby, Inc., an affiliate of Elsevier Inc. All rights reserved.

2. Identify the two major fluid compartments in the body and describe their composition.

3. Compare and contrast the causes and clinical manifestations of ECF volume excess and ECF volume deficit by completing the table below.

ECF Volume Imbalance	Causes	Clinical Manifestations
Fluid volume excess		
Fluid volume deficit		

Copyright © 2007 by Mosby, Inc., an affiliate of Elsevier Inc. All rights reserved.

4. Match each of the following terms related to fluid volume regulation with its corresponding definition.

Term	**Definition**
_____ Hydrostatic pressure	a. Movement of molecules from an area of high concentration to one of low concentration
_____ Oncotic pressure	
_____ Diffusion	b. Movement of water between two compartments separated by a membrane permeable to water but not to solutes; water moves from an area of low solute concentration (dilute) to one of high solute concentration (concentrated)
_____ Osmolarity	
_____ Aldosterone	
_____ Hypotonic	c. The force of pressure exerted by static water in a confined space—"water-pushing" pressure
_____ Osmosis	d. The total milliosmoles of solute per unit of total volume of solution (mOsm/L); pertains to fluids outside the body
_____ Antidiuretic hormone	
_____ Isotonic	e. The solid particle dissolved in a solution
_____ Solute	f. Any solution with a solute concentration equal to the osmolarity of normal body fluids or normal saline, about 300 mOsm/L
_____ Facilitated diffusion	
_____ Hypertonic	g. A hormone produced by the hypothalamus and released by the posterior pituitary gland to regulate body water
_____ Active transport	

h. Molecules combine with a specific carrier molecule to accelerate movement from an area of high concentration to one of low concentration

i. A hormone produced by the adrenal cortex that enhances sodium retention and potassium excretion

j. Process in which molecules move against the concentration gradient; requires energy

k. Any solution with a solute concentration (osmolarity) greater than that of normal body fluids (>310 mOsm/L)

l. The osmotic pressure exerted by colloids in solution; pulls fluid from the tissue space to the vascular space

m. Any solution with a solute concentration (osmolarity) less than that of normal body fluids (<270 mOsm/L)

Copyright © 2007 by Mosby, Inc., an affiliate of Elsevier Inc. All rights reserved.

Exercise 2

 CD-ROM Activity

 30 minutes

- Sign in to work at Pacific View Regional Hospital for Period of Care 1. (*Note:* If you are already in the virtual hospital from a previous exercise, click on **Leave the Floor** and then **Restart the Program** to get to the sign-in window.)
- From the Patient List, select Piya Jordan (Room 403).
- Click on **Go to Nurses' Station**.
- Click on **Chart** and then **403**.
- Click on **Emergency Department** and review this record.

  1. Record findings below that support the diagnosis of ECF volume deficit.

 • Click on **Nursing Admission**.

  2. Are there any additional findings noted on this document that support the diagnosis of ECF volume deficit? If so, list them below.

Copyright © 2007 by Mosby, Inc., an affiliate of Elsevier Inc. All rights reserved.

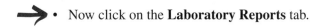 • Now click on the **Laboratory Reports** tab.

3. Record pertinent results below and describe the significance of each result in relation to the diagnosis of ECF volume deficit. (*Hint:* You may refer to your laboratory/diagnostic reference manual.)

4. An elevated serum sodium may occur with water loss or sodium gain. Which is occurring with Piya Jordan?

• Click on **History and Physical**.

5. What contributing factor(s) led to this fluid imbalance?

• Now click on **Physician's Orders** and read the initial orders for Piya Jordan.

6. Identify orders that are appropriate management strategies for the treatment of ECF volume deficit and write your findings below.

Copyright © 2007 by Mosby, Inc., an affiliate of Elsevier Inc. All rights reserved.

7. Develop an appropriate plan of care for Piya Jordan related to management of her fluid volume deficit.

Collaborative Plan of Care	ECF Volume Deficit
Patient outcomes	
Assessment parameters	
Collaborative care interventions	

Exercise 3

 CD-ROM Activity

 45 minutes

- Sign in to work at Pacific View Regional Hospital for Period of Care 1. (*Note:* If you are already in the virtual hospital from a previous exercise, click on **Leave the Floor** and then **Restart the Program** to get to the sign-in window.)
- From the Patient List, select Patricia Newman (Room 406).
- Click on **Go to Nurses' Station**.
- Click on **Chart** and then **406**.
- Read the **Emergency Department** record.

1. Identify assessment findings related to fluid balance and record below. How do these findings differ from those for Piya Jordan? Are there any similarities?

Copyright © 2007 by Mosby, Inc., an affiliate of Elsevier Inc. All rights reserved.

→ • Click on **Nursing Admission**.

    2. Are there any additional findings noted on this document related to fluid balance and/or imbalance? If so, list them below. How do they compare with findings for Piya Jordan?

→ • Now review the **Laboratory Results**.

    3. Record pertinent results below and describe the significance of each result in relation to fluid balance. Describe any differences between these findings and those for Piya Jordan.

    4. Based on your findings, does Patricia Newman have a fluid imbalance? If so, what type?

    5. What are the contributing factors for this patient's potential or actual fluid imbalance?

Copyright © 2007 by Mosby, Inc., an affiliate of Elsevier Inc. All rights reserved.

➤ • Read Patricia Newman's **History and Physical**.

6. What coexisting illness might have an impact on the selection and rate of IV fluid therapy?

7. Develop an appropriate plan of care for patients with ECF volume excess by completing the chart below.

Collaborative Plan of Care	**ECF Volume Excess**
Patient outcomes	
Assessment parameters	
Collaborative care interventions	

Copyright © 2007 by Mosby, Inc., an affiliate of Elsevier Inc. All rights reserved.

Electrolyte Imbalances, Part 1—Potassium

 Reading Assignment: Fluid, Electrolyte, and Acid-Base Imbalances (Chapter 17)

Patients: Piya Jordan, Room 403
Patricia Newman, Room 406

Goal: Utilize the nursing process to competently care for patients with electrolyte imbalances.

Objectives:

1. Describe normal physiologic influences on electrolyte balance.
2. Identify specific etiologic factors related to hypokalemia for assigned patients.
3. Research potential drug interactions related to hypokalemia for assigned patients.
4. Assess patients for clinical manifestations related to hypo- and hyperkalemia.
5. Utilize the nursing process to correctly administer IV potassium chloride per physician orders.

In this lesson you will assess, plan, and implement care for two patients with hypokalemia. Piya Jordan is a 68-year-old female admitted with nausea and vomiting for several days following weeks of poor appetite and increasing weakness. Patricia Newman is a 61-year-old female admitted with pneumonia and a history of emphysema for 12 years. Begin this activity by reviewing the general functions of electrolytes within the body as presented in your textbook. Answer the following questions to cement your understanding of the normal physiologic concepts related to potassium balance.

Exercise 1

 Clinical Preparation: Writing Activity

20 minutes

1. Define the following terms.

   a. Ion

Copyright © 2007 by Mosby, Inc., an affiliate of Elsevier Inc. All rights reserved.

   b. Cation

   c. Anion

   d. Valence

2. Identify the following electrolytes.

   a. Primary ICF cation

   b. Primary ICF anion

   c. Primary ECF cation

   d. Primary ECF anion

3. Identify the functions of potassium within the body.

4. Describe the physiologic influences on potassium balance.

Copyright © 2007 by Mosby, Inc., an affiliate of Elsevier Inc. All rights reserved.

Exercise 3

 CD-ROM Activity

 30 minutes

- Sign in to work at Pacific View Regional Hospital for Period of Care 1. (*Note:* If you are already in the virtual hospital from a previous exercise, click on **Leave the Floor** and then **Restart the Program** to get to the sign-in window.)
- From the Patient List, select Patricia Newman (Room 406).
- Click on **Go to Nurses' Station**.
- Click on **Chart** and then **406**.
- Click on **Laboratory Reports**.

   1. What was Patricia Newman's initial potassium level this morning?

- Click on **History and Physical**.

   2. What would be the most likely cause for hypokalemia in this patient?

- Click on **Physician's Orders**.

   3. What did the physician order to treat this electrolyte imbalance?

- Click on **Return to Nurses' Station**.
- Click on **MAR** and then **406**.

   4. What is missing from this order?

Copyright © 2007 by Mosby, Inc., an affiliate of Elsevier Inc. All rights reserved.

5. Where could you verify this missing information?

6. What is the difference between the treatment of hypokalemia for Piya Jordan and that for Patricia Newman? Provide a rationale for the difference.

→ • Click on **Return to Nurses' Station**.
  • Click on **Chart** and then **406**.
  • Click on **Physician's Orders**.

7. Look again at the physician's orders. Is there an order for any follow-up lab work?

8. What is the nurse's responsibility in regard to follow-up lab work? How would you handle this situation?

→ • Click on **Return to Nurses' Station**.
  • Click on **406** to go to Patricia Newman's room.
  • Select **Patient Care** and then **Nurse-Client Interactions**.
  • Select and view the video titled **0740: Evaluation—Response to Care**. (*Note:* Check the virtual clock to see whether enough time has elapsed. You can use the fast-forward feature to advance the time by 2-minute intervals if the video is not yet available. Then click on **Patient Care** and **Nurse-Client Interactions** to refresh the screen.)

Copyright © 2007 by Mosby, Inc., an affiliate of Elsevier Inc. All rights reserved.

9. Although Patricia Newman is happy that her chest does not hurt like it did, what does she verbalize as a concern?

10. What is the nurse's response to the patient's expressed concern?

11. When evaluating the care of Patricia Newman, for what potential complications of IV potassium therapy would you monitor? (*Hint:* Consult the Drug Guide by clicking on the **Drug** icon in the lower left corner of your screen.)

Copyright © 2007 by Mosby, Inc., an affiliate of Elsevier Inc. All rights reserved.

Electrolyte Imbalances, Part 2—Calcium, Phosphate, and Sodium

✐ **Reading Assignment:** Fluid, Electrolyte, and Acid-Base Imbalances (Chapter 17)

Patient: Pablo Rodriguez, Room 405

Goal: Utilize the nursing process to competently care for patients with electrolyte imbalances.

Objectives:

1. Describe the pathophysiologic basis of electrolyte imbalances noted on a specific patient.
2. Identify specific etiologic factor(s) related to hypercalcemia, hyponatremia, and hypophosphatemia in the assigned patient.
3. Assess the assigned patient for clinical manifestations related to sodium, calcium, and phosphate imbalances.
4. Describe nursing interventions appropriate when caring for a patient with hypercalcemia, hyponatremia, and hypophosphatemia.
5. Evaluate the effectiveness of medication prescribed to treat electrolyte imbalances.

In this lesson you will assess, plan, and implement care for a patient with several electrolyte imbalances. Pablo Rodriguez is a 71-year-old male who is admitted with nausea and vomiting for several days. He has a 1-year history of lung carcinoma. Begin this activity by reviewing the general functions of specific electrolytes within the body as presented in your textbook. Answer the questions on the following page to cement your understanding of the normal physiologic concepts related to phosphorous, sodium, chloride, and calcium balance.

Copyright © 2007 by Mosby, Inc., an affiliate of Elsevier Inc. All rights reserved.

Exercise 1

Clinical Preparation: Writing Activity

15 minutes

1. Prior to caring for a patient with multiple electrolyte imbalances, it is imperative that you first review and reinforce general concepts related to specific electrolytes. Using the textbook, complete the table below by providing information related to calcium, phosphorus, and sodium. Refer to this table as you proceed through the CD-ROM activities to relate textbook knowledge to actual patient care.

Electrolyte	Normal Level	Functions	Major Location	Pathophysiologic Influences
Calcium				
Phosphorus				
Sodium				

Copyright © 2007 by Mosby, Inc., an affiliate of Elsevier Inc. All rights reserved.

Exercise 2

 CD-ROM Activity

 45 minutes

- Sign in to work at Pacific View Regional Hospital for Period of Care 1. (*Note:* If you are already in the virtual hospital from a previous exercise, click on **Leave the Floor** and then **Restart the Program** to get to the sign-in window.)
- From the Patient List, select Pablo Rodriguez (Room 405).
- Click on **Go to Nurses' Station**.
- Click on **Chart** and then **405**.
- Click on **Laboratory Reports**.

1. Complete the table below by recording Pablo Rodriguez's serum chemistry results. Identify abnormal values by marking as H (for high) or L (for low).

Lab Test	Lab Result Tuesday 2000	Lab Result Wednesday 0730
Sodium		
Potassium		
Chloride		
Calcium		
Phosphorus		
Magnesium		

 - Click on **Emergency Department** and review this record.

2. What would be the most likely cause for the hyponatremia noted on admission for this patient?

Copyright © 2007 by Mosby, Inc., an affiliate of Elsevier Inc. All rights reserved.

3. Hyponatremia can be associated with both hypovolemia (actual sodium loss) and hypervolemia (excessive water gain). Initially, in the ED, what do you think Pablo Rodriguez's volume status was? Explain.

4. Because GI losses of sodium are accompanied by greater or equal loss of water, explain what causes the lower serum sodium concentration.

5. What did the physician order to treat this electrolyte imbalance?

6. Find Pablo Rodriguez's sodium level for Wednesday at 0730. Was the physician's ordered treatment effective? Can you anticipate or suggest any changes in orders?

→ • Click on **Return to Nurses' Station**.
   • Click on **EPR** and then **Login**.
   • Select **405** as the patient and **Intake and Output** as the category.

7. Record the I&O shift totals for Pablo Rodriguez below.

Shift Totals	Tuesday 0705	Tuesday 1505	Tuesday 2305	Wednesday 0705
Intake				
Output				

Copyright © 2007 by Mosby, Inc., an affiliate of Elsevier Inc. All rights reserved.

8. Based on the above I&O totals obtained after the patient received IV replacement therapy, what factor(s) may be contributing to the persistant hyponatremia? Explain.

9. What other lab tests might be useful to more accurately determine the patient's hydration status? (*Hint:* See page 338 in your textbook.)

• Click on **Return to Nurses' Station**.
• Click on **405**.
• Select **Patient Care**.

10. Complete a physical assessment on Pablo Rodriguez, specifically looking for clinical manifestations of hyponatremia. (*Hint:* See pages 325-326 in your textbook.) Document your findings in the table below and on the next page; underline or highlight the manifestations that correlate with hyponatremia.

Areas Assessed	Findings on Physical Examination
Cardiovascular	
Respiratory	

Copyright © 2007 by Mosby, Inc., an affiliate of Elsevier Inc. All rights reserved.

Areas Assessed	Findings on Physical Examination
Neuromuscular	
Gastrointestinal	

➡ • Click on **Chart**.
• Click on **Nursing Admission**.

11. What other factors could be causing or contributing to the manifestations that you underlined or highlighted in the table in question 10?

12. Based on your answers to questions 10 and 11, what conclusion can you make regarding these clinical manifestations and Pablo Rodriguez's sodium levels?

 13. What additional clinical manifestations of hyponatremia might you expect to find in other patients with this electrolyte imbalance accompanied by hypovolemia? (*Hint:* See pages 321-326 in your textbook.)

Copyright © 2007 by Mosby, Inc., an affiliate of Elsevier Inc. All rights reserved.

14. How would these clinical manifestations differ if the patient's fluid volume status was normal or increased?

15. If Pablo Rodriguez's sodium level were 120 (severe hyponatremia), how would the treatment differ?

Exercise 3

 CD-ROM Activity

 60 minutes

- Sign in to work at Pacific View Regional Hospital for Period of Care 3. (*Note:* If you are already in the virtual hospital from a previous exercise, click on **Leave the Floor** and then **Restart the Program** to get to the sign-in window.)
- From the Patient List, select Pablo Rodriguez (Room 405).
- Click on **Go to Nurses' Station**.
- Click on **Chart** and then **405**.
- Click on **History and Physical**.

1. What electrolyte imbalances did Pablo Rodriguez present with on admission?

 • Click on **Laboratory Reports**.

2. What was Pablo Rodriguez's calcium level on admission to the ED on Tuesday evening?

Copyright © 2007 by Mosby, Inc., an affiliate of Elsevier Inc. All rights reserved.

3. How does this level correlate with the physician's diagnosis? Speculate as to the reason for the discrepancy.

4. What was Pablo Rodriguez's phosphorus level during the same time frame?

5. How does this relate to his calcium level? Explain the pathophysiologic rationale supporting your answer.

6. What other laboratory test(s) would give the nurse a more accurate picture of Pablo Rodriguez's calcium balance? Explain your answer.

➡ • Click on **History and Physical**.

7. What would be the most likely cause for hypercalcemia in this patient? (*Hint:* See Table 17-8 in your textbook.)

➡ • Click on **Physician's Orders**.

Copyright © 2007 by Mosby, Inc., an affiliate of Elsevier Inc. All rights reserved.

8. What medication did the ED physician order to treat the hypercalcemia?

9. Describe the mechanism of action of the above medication.

10. Plicamycin can also be used to treat hypercalcemia. Why did the physician choose pamidronate over plicamycin? (*Hint:* See page 330 in your textbook.)

→ • Click on **Return to Nurses' Station**.
   • Click on the **Drug Guide** on the counter.

11. What nursing assessments are appropriate related to the administration of pamidronate?

→ • Click on **Return to Nurses' Station**.
   • Click on **Chart** and then **405**.
   • Click on **Laboratory Reports**.

Copyright © 2007 by Mosby, Inc., an affiliate of Elsevier Inc. All rights reserved.

12. What were Pablo Rodriguez's calcium and phosphorus levels this morning (Wednesday at 0730)?

13. Was the prescribed medication effective? Is the patient out of danger?

➡ • Click on **Return to Nurses' Station**.
  • Click on **Kardex** and then on tab **405**.

14. What intravenous fluids is Pablo Rodriguez receiving?

15. What is the purpose of IV hydration in relation to serum calcium levels?

16. Is this the solution you would normally expect to administer to a patient with hypercalcemia? If not, what solution would you expect?

➡ • Click on **Return to Nurses' Station**.
  • Click on **MAR** and then on tab **405**.

17. What medication is scheduled to be administered at 1500?

Copyright © 2007 by Mosby, Inc., an affiliate of Elsevier Inc. All rights reserved.

18. What electrolyte imbalance will this medication correct? Explain your answer. (*Hint:* For help, consult the Drug Guide.)

19. What nursing assessments must be completed before this drug is administered?

20. Do you have any concerns regarding administering this drug at this specific time? (*Hint:* Check the patient's GI history on admission.)

→ • Click on **Return to Nurses' Station**.
  • Click on **405** to go to the patient's room.
  • Click on **Patient Care**.

21. Complete a physical assessment on Pablo Rodriguez (including vital signs.) Document your findings below and on the next page.

Areas Assessed	Findings on Physical Examination
Cardiovascular	
Respiratory	

Copyright © 2007 by Mosby, Inc., an affiliate of Elsevier Inc. All rights reserved.

Areas Assessed	**Findings on Physical Examination**
Neuromuscular	
Gastrointestinal	

22. Is Pablo Rodriguez demonstrating any clinical manifestations of hypercalcemia? If yes, describe the pathophysiologic basis for the symptoms. If not, explain why not.

23. If Pablo Rodriguez's calcium level were 12.5, what other clinical manifestations might the nurse expect to find? (*Hint:* See pages 329-331 in your textbook.)

24. When evaluating this patient's renal output, what potential complication of hypercalcemia would you be alert for?

25. After successful treatment of Pablo Rodriguez, the nurse must be alert for overcorrecting of the electrolyte imbalance. For what clinical manifestations should the nurse monitor this patient related to hypocalcemia and hyperphosphatemia?

Copyright © 2007 by Mosby, Inc., an affiliate of Elsevier Inc. All rights reserved.

Acid-Base Imbalance

Reading Assignment: Fluid, Electrolyte, and Acid-Base Imbalances (Chapter 17)

Patients: Jacquline Catanazaro, Room 402
Patricia Newman, Room 406

Goal: Utilize the nursing process to competently care for patients with acid-base imbalances.

Objectives:

1. Describe the pathophysiologic basis of acid-base imbalance noted in assigned patients.
2. Identify specific etiologic factor(s) related to respiratory acidosis in the assigned patients.
3. Assess the assigned patients for clinical manifestations related to respiratory acidosis.
4. Describe nursing interventions appropriate when caring for specific patients with respiratory acidosis.
5. Evaluate the effectiveness of medication prescribed to treat acid-base imbalances.

In this lesson you will assess, plan, and implement care for patients with acid-base imbalance. Jacquline Catanazaro is a 45-year-old female admitted with exacerbation of asthma and schizophrenia. Patricia Newman is a 61-year-old female admitted with pneumonia and a history of emphysema for 12 years. Begin this lesson by reviewing the general concepts of acid-base balance as presented in your textbook.

Exercise 1

 Clinical Preparation: Writing Activity

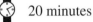 20 minutes

1. Define the following terms.

    a. Acid

Copyright © 2007 by Mosby, Inc., an affiliate of Elsevier Inc. All rights reserved.

b. Base

c. pH

2. Describe three methods of acid-base homeostasis by completing the following table.

	Type of Defense	Mechanisms of Action
First Line of Defense: Reacts immediately		
Second Line of Defense: Reacts within minutes		
Third Line of Defense: Takes 2-3 days to respond maximally		

Exercise 2

 CD-ROM Activity

 45 minutes

- Sign in to work at Pacific View Regional Hospital for Period of Care 1. (*Note:* If you are already in the virtual hospital from a previous exercise, click on **Leave the Floor** and then **Restart the Program** to get to the sign-in window.)
- From the Patient List, select Jacquline Catanazaro (Room 402).
- Click on **Go to Nurses' Station**.
- Click on **Chart** and then **402**.
- Click on **History and Physical**.

Copyright © 2007 by Mosby, Inc., an affiliate of Elsevier Inc. All rights reserved.

1. Is there anything in Jacquline Catanazaro's history that would put her at risk for an acid-base imbalance?

 • Click on **Return to Nurses' Station**.
• Click on **402** to go to the patient's room.
• Click on **Patient Care** and then **Nurse-Client Interactions**.
• Select and view the video titled **0730: Intervention—Airway**. (*Note:* Check the virtual clock to see whether enough time has elapsed. You can use the fast-forward feature to advance the time by 2-minute intervals if the video is not yet available. Then click on **Patient Care** and **Nurse-Client Interactions** to refresh the screen.)

2. Based on Jacquline Catanazaro's history, what would you expect to be causing her respiratory distress?

3. Why is the nurse waiting until the ABGs are being drawn to give the patient a nebulizer treatment?

 • Click on **Chart** and then **402**.
• Click on **Laboratory Reports**.

4. What are the results of Jacquline Catanazaro's two most recent ABGs? Record them below.

ABGs	Monday 1030	Wednesday 0730
pH		
PaO$_2$		
PaCO$_2$		
O$_2$ sat		
Bicarb		

Copyright © 2007 by Mosby, Inc., an affiliate of Elsevier Inc. All rights reserved.

5. How would you interpret the results in question 4? Is the acid-base imbalance compensated or uncompensated (fully or partially)? Explain your answer.

6. Since this patient's respiratory difficulties are of an acute nature, what acid-base regulation mechanisms would you expect to be working to compensate for her respiratory acidosis?

7. Based on Jacquline Catanazaro's medical diagnosis, what is the underlying pathophysiological problem leading to the respiratory acidosis?

→ • Click on **Return to Room 402**.
 • Click on **Patient Care**.

8. Perform a complete physical assessment on the patient and record your findings below and on the next page.

Areas Assessed	Findings on Physical Examination
Neurologic	

Copyright © 2007 by Mosby, Inc., an affiliate of Elsevier Inc. All rights reserved.

Areas Assessed	**Findings on Physical Examination**
Musculoskeletal	
Cardiovascular	
Respiratory	
Integumentary	

9. Does this patient have any clinical manifestations of respiratory acidosis? If so, please describe. If not, how do you explain?

→ • Click on **Take Vital Signs**.

10. What is Jacquline Catanazaro's respiratory rate? How does this correlate with her asthma and respiratory acidosis?

Copyright © 2007 by Mosby, Inc., an affiliate of Elsevier Inc. All rights reserved.

11. If Jacquline Catanazaro's pH were 7.2, how might her physical assessment differ? Document the expected clinical manifestations of respiratory acidosis below.

Areas Assessed	Expected Findings on Physical Examination
Neurologic	
Cardiovascular	
Gastrointestinal	
Neuromuscular	
Respiratory	

→ • Click on **Chart** and then **402**.
 • Click on **Physician's Orders**.

Copyright © 2007 by Mosby, Inc., an affiliate of Elsevier Inc. All rights reserved.

12. Look at the most recent physician's orders. What medication is ordered to treat the respiratory acidosis? What is the medication's underlying mechanism of action to correct the acidosis?

- Click on **Return to Room 402**.
- Click on **Leave the Floor** and then **Restart the Program**.
- Sign in for Period of Care 2.
- From the Patient List, select Jacquline Catanazaro (Room 402).
- Click on **Go to Nurses' Station**.
- Click on **Chart** and then **402**.
- Click on **Laboratory Reports**.

13. Interpret the ABGs drawn at 1000. Was the treatment effective?

Exercise 3

 CD-ROM Activity

 45 minutes

- Sign in to work at Pacific View Regional Hospital for Period of Care 1. (*Note:* If you are already in the virtual hospital from a previous exercise, click on **Leave the Floor** and then **Restart the Program** to get to the sign-in window.)
- From the Patient List, select Patricia Newman (Room 406).
- Click on **Go to Nurses' Station**.
- Click on **Chart** and then **406**.
- Click on **History and Physical**.

1. Is there anything in Patricia Newman's history that would put her at risk for an acid-base imbalance? If so, what?

Copyright © 2007 by Mosby, Inc., an affiliate of Elsevier Inc. All rights reserved.

➡ • Click on **Laboratory Reports**.

2. What are the results of Patricia Newman's two most recent ABGs? Document your findings below.

ABGs	Tuesday 2300	Wednesday 0500
pH		
PaO$_2$		
PaCO$_2$		
O$_2$ sat		
Bicarb		

3. How would you interpret the above results? Is the acid-base imbalance compensated or uncompensated (fully or partially)? Explain your answer.

4. Based on the chronic aspect of Patricia Newman's respiratory difficulties, what compensatory mechanisms would you expect to be working to correct the respiratory acidosis?

5. Based on the ABG results, has her condition improved or worsened since admission?

Copyright © 2007 by Mosby, Inc., an affiliate of Elsevier Inc. All rights reserved.

• Click on **Return to Room 406**.
  • Click on **Chart**.
  • Click on **Nurse's Notes**.

6. Read the notes for Wednesday 0730. Describe the actions taken by the nurse. Are they appropriate or not? Explain your answer.

7. What additional actions do you think would be appropriate at this time?

 • Click on **Laboratory Reports**.
  8. What is the patient's serum potassium level?

9. Hyperkalemia is frequently associated with acidosis as potassium moves out of the cell to compensate for hydrogen moving into the cell. How, then, would you explain the patient's hypokalemia occurring along with respiratory acidosis? (*Hint:* Check the concurrent medications.)

10. Based on Patricia Newman's medical diagnosis, what is the underlying pathophysiological problem leading to her respiratory acidosis? (*Hint:* Refer to Chapters 28 and 29 of your textbook.) How does this differ from Jacquline Catanazaro's problem in Exercise 2?

Copyright © 2007 by Mosby, Inc., an affiliate of Elsevier Inc. All rights reserved.

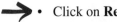 • Click on **Return to Room 406**.
• Click on **Patient Care**.

11. Perform a complete physical assessment, including vital signs, on Patricia Newman. Document your findings below.

Areas Assessed	Findings on Physical Examination
Neurologic	
Musculoskeletal	
Cardiovascular	
Respiratory	
Integumentary	

Copyright © 2007 by Mosby, Inc., an affiliate of Elsevier Inc. All rights reserved.

12. Does Patricia Newman have any clinical manifestations of respiratory acidosis? If so, please describe. If not, explain why not.

 13. What nursing interventions could you, as a graduate nurse, plan and implement to improve Patricia Newman's acid-base balance and prevent complications? (*Hint:* Again refer to textbook Chapters 28 and 29 for disease-specific interventions.)

Copyright © 2007 by Mosby, Inc., an affiliate of Elsevier Inc. All rights reserved.

LESSON **10** ─────────────────

Perioperative Care

Reading Assignment: Nursing Management: Preoperative Care (Chapter 18)
Nursing Management: Postoperative Care (Chapter 20)

Patients: Piya Jordan, Room 403
Clarence Hughes, Room 404

Goal: Utilize the nursing process to competently care for perioperative patients.

Objectives:

1. Document a complete history and physical on a preoperative patient.
2. Identify appropriate rationales for preoperative orders on an assigned patient.
3. Evaluate completeness of preoperative teaching on a patient scheduled for surgery.
4. Document a focused assessment for a patient transferred from PACU to a medical-surgical unit.
5. Plan appropriate interventions to prevent postoperative complications in an assigned patient.
6. Utilize the nursing process to correctly administer scheduled and prn medications to an assigned patient.

In this lesson you will learn the essentials of caring for patients in both the preoperative and postoperative stages of surgery. You will document, assess, plan, implement, and evaluate care given. Piya Jordan is a 68-year-old female admitted with nausea and vomiting for 3 days. Clarence Hughes is a 73-year-old male admitted for an elective knee replacement.

Exercise 1

 CD-ROM Activity

 40 minutes

- Sign in to work at Pacific View Regional Hospital for Period of Care 1. (*Note:* If you are already in the virtual hospital from a previous exercise, click on **Leave the Floor** and then **Restart the Program** to get to the sign-in window.)
- From the Patient List, select Piya Jordan (Room 403).
- Click on **Go to Nurses' Station**.
- Click on **Chart** and then **403**.
- Click on **Emergency Department**.

139

Copyright © 2007 by Mosby, Inc., an affiliate of Elsevier Inc. All rights reserved.

1. What day and time did Piya Jordan arrive in the Emergency Department?

2. What complaints (problems) brought her to the ED?

3. What were her primary and secondary admitting diagnoses?

→ • Click on **Nursing Admission**.

4. Important areas of data collection for the health history during the preoperative period are listed below and on the next two pages. Using the Nursing Admission form as your source, record the data collected for each area. If an area was not completed, write "No data." (*Hint:* See pages 344-350 in your textbook for clarification of each section.)

Areas of Data Collection	Piya Jordan's Data
Psychosocial assessment	
Past health history	
Prior surgical procedures	
Prior experience with anesthesia	
Family history	

Copyright © 2007 by Mosby, Inc., an affiliate of Elsevier Inc. All rights reserved.

Areas of Data Collection	Piya Jordan's Data
Current medications (including use of herbs and dietary supplements)	
Allergies (including sensitivity to latex products)	
Review of Systems Cardiovascular	
Respiratory	
Nervous	
Urinary	
Gastrointestinal	
Hepatic	
Integumentary	
Musculoskeletal	
Endocrine	
Immune	

Copyright © 2007 by Mosby, Inc., an affiliate of Elsevier Inc. All rights reserved.

Areas of Data Collection	Piya Jordan's Data
Fluid and electrolyte	
Nutritional status	
Functional Health Patterns Health Perception—Health Management Pattern	
Nutritional-Metabolic Pattern	
Elimination Pattern	
Activity-Exercise Pattern	
Sleep-Rest Pattern	
Cognitive-Perceptual Pattern	
Self-Perception/Self-Concept Pattern	
Role-Relationship Pattern	
Sexuality-Reproductive Pattern	
Coping-Stress Tolerance Pattern	
Value-Belief Pattern	

Copyright © 2007 by Mosby, Inc., an affiliate of Elsevier Inc. All rights reserved.

• Click on **History and Physical**.

 5. In addition to data obtained from the health history, a physical examination provides necessary and important data for the preoperative assessment. For each of the areas listed below, identify in the middle column the key items to assess (excluding history and lab results) according to your textbook (pages 347-349). In the last column, document the results from the physician's assessment as noted in the H&P. If an area was not completed, write "No data."

Physical Examination Area	Key Specific Assessments from Textbook	Results for Piya Jordan
Cardiovascular		
Respiratory		
Neurologic		
Urinary		
Hepatic		
Integumentary		
Musculoskeletal		
Gastrointestinal		

Copyright © 2007 by Mosby, Inc., an affiliate of Elsevier Inc. All rights reserved.

→ • Click on **Laboratory Reports**.

6. The most common preoperative diagnostic tests are listed below. For each test, record results for Piya Jordan. If a test was not completed, write "No data."

Diagnostic Tests	Piya Jordan's Results
CBC	
WBC	
RBC	
Hemoglobin	
Hematocrit	
Platelets	
Electrolytes	
Glucose	
Sodium	
Potassium	
Chloride	
CO_2	
Creatinine	
BUN	
Coagulation Tests	
PTT	
PT	
INR	
Urinalysis	
ABGs	
Liver Function Tests	
Bilirubin (total)	
Protein	
Albumin	
Alkaline phosphates	
ALT (SGPT)	
AST (SGOT)	
Type and Crossmatch	

Copyright © 2007 by Mosby, Inc., an affiliate of Elsevier Inc. All rights reserved.

7. Are any of Piya Jordan's lab results abnormal or of concern for a patient preparing to undergo surgery? Explain.

Exercise 2

 CD-ROM Activity

 30 minutes

- Sign in to work at Pacific View Regional Hospital for Period of Care 1. (*Note:* If you are already in the virtual hospital from a previous exercise, click on **Leave the Floor** and then **Restart the Program** to get to the sign-in window.)
- From the Patient List, select Piya Jordan (Room 403).
- Click on **Go to Nurses' Station**.
- Click on **Chart** and then **403**.
- Click on the **Consents** tab.

1. For what procedure(s) has Piya Jordan given written consent?

2. Who signed the consent form as the witness?

3. Who is responsible for providing detailed information about the procedure(s) for which the patient has given consent?

4. What is the nurse's responsibility in regard to obtaining informed consent?

Copyright © 2007 by Mosby, Inc., an affiliate of Elsevier Inc. All rights reserved.

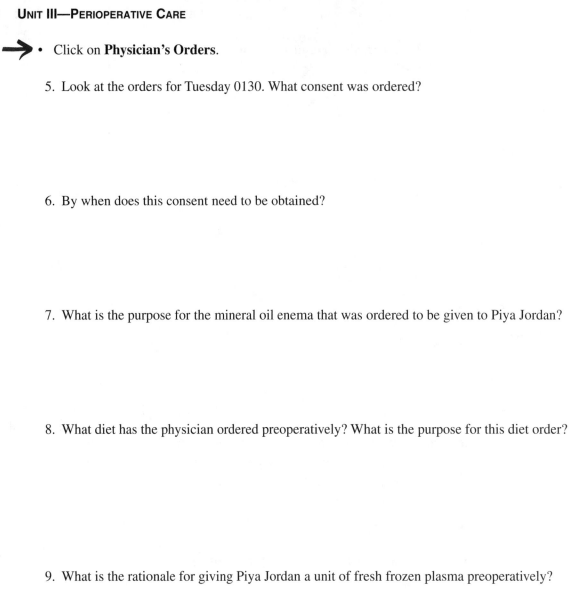

→ • Click on **Physician's Orders**.

5. Look at the orders for Tuesday 0130. What consent was ordered?

6. By when does this consent need to be obtained?

7. What is the purpose for the mineral oil enema that was ordered to be given to Piya Jordan?

8. What diet has the physician ordered preoperatively? What is the purpose for this diet order?

9. What is the rationale for giving Piya Jordan a unit of fresh frozen plasma preoperatively?

10. What is the rationale for ordering a dose of cefotetan on call to the OR? Is this a safe order to administer to Piya Jordan? Explain why or why not.

Copyright © 2007 by Mosby, Inc., an affiliate of Elsevier Inc. All rights reserved.

• Click on **Surgical Reports**.

11. Scroll down to the Preoperative Patient Instruction Sheet. What preoperative teaching was completed?

12. Scroll down further to the Preoperative Checklist. What additional teaching was given to Piya Jordan prior to admission?

13. What process information should be explained to Piya Jordan's family? (*Hint:* See Table 18-7 in your textbook.)

Exercise 3

 CD-ROM Activity

 45 minutes

Clarence Hughes' scheduled surgery is now complete. You will be reviewing care provided to him immediately postop, as well as planning and evaluating care given during this time period.

• Sign in to work at Pacific View Regional Hospital for Period of Care 1. (*Note:* If you are already in the virtual hospital from a previous exercise, click on **Leave the Floor** and then **Restart the Program** to get to the sign-in window.)
• From the Patient List, select Clarence Hughes (Room 404).
• Click on **Go to Nurses' Station**.
• Click on **EPR** and then **Login**.
• Select **404** as the patient.
• Review the Vital Signs, Respiratory, Neurologic, Integumentary, IV, Wounds and Drains, Excretory, and any other EPR categories necessary to answer the following question.

Copyright © 2007 by Mosby, Inc., an affiliate of Elsevier Inc. All rights reserved.

1. On arrival to the medical-surgical clinical unit, a postoperative patient requires an immediate focused assessment. For each area specified in the left column below, document the assessment findings recorded by the nurse on Sunday at 1600 when Clarence Hughes arrived on the medical-surgical clinical unit.

Focused Assessment Areas	Clarence Hughes' Assessment Findings
Airway	
Breathing	
Neuropsychologic status	
Wound, dressing, and drainage tubes	
Vital signs	
Intravenous fluids	
Color and appearance of skin	
Urinary status	

Copyright © 2007 by Mosby, Inc., an affiliate of Elsevier Inc. All rights reserved.

2. How would you analyze Clarence Hughes' blood pressure and heart rate noted in the previous question? What actions should be taken? How often should vital signs be monitored? (*Hint:* See page 386 in your textbook.)

3. At what point would you notify the surgeon regarding Clarence Hughes' vital signs?

 • Still in the EPR, select **Intake and Output** as the category.

4. In the table below, record Clarence Hughes' I&O for the past 3 days at the times specified.

	Sun 1500-2300	Mon 2300-0700	Mon 0700-1500	Mon 1500-2300	Tues 2300-0700	Tues 0700-1500	Tues 1500-2300	Wed 2300-0700
Intake								
Output								

5. Which is greater—Clarence Hughes' intake or output? By how much? Is this expected?

6. What are the possible consequences if this trend in fluid balance continues?

Copyright © 2007 by Mosby, Inc., an affiliate of Elsevier Inc. All rights reserved.

→ • Click on **Exit EPR**.
  • Click on **Chart** and then **404**.
  • Click on **Physician's Orders**.

7. Look at the physician's postoperative orders written on Sunday at 1600. What is ordered to prevent postoperative atelectasis?

8. What additional interventions can you suggest to further prevent atelectasis?

9. What is ordered to prevent DVT?

10. Scroll up to look at the orders for Monday 0715. What did the physician order at this time to prevent DVT postoperatively?

11. What additional interventions can you suggest to further prevent DVT?

12. What wound care is ordered on Sunday?

13. At what point may the dressing be removed and the incision left open to air?

Copyright © 2007 by Mosby, Inc., an affiliate of Elsevier Inc. All rights reserved.

• Click on **Return to Room 404**.

- Inside Clarence Hughes' room, click on **Take Vital Signs**. Review these results.
- Next, click on **Clinical Alerts**.
- Now select **Patient Care** and then **Nurse-Client Interactions**.
- Select and view the video titled **0735: Empathy**. (*Note:* Check the virtual clock to see whether enough time has elapsed. You can use the fast-forward feature to advance the time by 2-minute intervals if the video is not yet available. Then click on **Patient Care** and **Nurse-Client Interactions** to refresh the screen.)

14. What is Clarence Hughes' major concern at this point?

 • Now click on **Medication Room**.

- From the Medication Room, click on **MAR** to determine medications that Clarence Hughes is ordered to receive at 0800 and any appropriate prn medications you may want to administer. (*Note:* You may click on **Review MAR** at any time to verify the correct medication order. Remember to look at the patient name on the MAR to make sure you have the correct patient's record—you must click on the correct room number within the MAR. Click on **Return to Medication Room** after reviewing the correct MAR.)
- Click on **Unit Dosage** at the top of your screen or on the Unit Dosage cabinet to the right of Automated System.
- From the close-up view of the Unit Dosage drawers, click on drawer **404**.
- From the list of available medications in the top window, select the medication(s) you would like to administer. After each medication you select, click on **Put Medication on Tray**.
- When you have finished putting your selected medications on the tray, click on **Close Drawer**.
- Click on **View Medication Room**.
- This time, click on **Automated System** (or on the Automated System unit itself). Your name and password will automatically appear. Click on **Login**.
- In box 1, select the correct patient; in box 2, choose the appropriate Automated System Drawer for this patient. Then click on **Open Drawer**.
- From the list of available medications, select the medication(s) you would like to administer. For each one selected, click on **Put Medication on Tray**. When you are finished, click on **Close Drawer**.
- Click **View Medication Room**.
- From the Medication Room, click on **Preparation** (or on the preparation tray on the counter); then highlight the medication you want to administer. Click on **Prepare**.
- Provide any information requested by the Preparation Wizard.
- Click **Next**, choose the correct patient to administer this medication to, and click **Finish**.
- Repeat the previous two steps until you have prepared all the medications you want to administer.
- You can click **Review Your Medications** and then **Return to Medication Room** when you are ready. Once you are back in the Medication Room, you can go directly to Clarence Hughes' room by clicking on **404** at the bottom of the screen.

Copyright © 2007 by Mosby, Inc., an affiliate of Elsevier Inc. All rights reserved.

- Administer the medication, utilizing the five rights of medication administration. After you have collected the appropriate assessment data and are ready for administration, click **Patient Care** and then **Medication Administration**. Verify that the correct patient and medication(s) appear in the left-hand window. Then click the down arrow next to Select. From the drop-down menu, select **Administer** and complete the Administration Wizard by providing any information requested. When the Wizard stops asking for information, click **Administer to Patient**. Specify **Yes** when asked whether this administration should be recorded in the MAR. Finally, click **Finish**.

Now let's see how you did!

- Click on **Leave the Floor** at the bottom of your screen.
- From the Floor Menu, select **Look at Your Preceptor's Evaluation**.
- Click on **Medication Scorecard**.

15. Note below whether or not you correctly administered the appropriate medication(s). If not, why do you think you were incorrect? According to Table C in this scorecard, what resources should be used and what important assessments should be completed before administering the medication(s)? Did you utilize these resources and perform these assessments correctly?

Copyright © 2007 by Mosby, Inc., an affiliate of Elsevier Inc. All rights reserved.

LESSON **11**

Glaucoma

 Reading Assignment: Nursing Management: Visual and Auditory Problems
(Chapter 22)

Patient: Clarence Hughes, Room 404

Goal: Utilize the nursing process to competently care for patients with glaucoma.

Objectives:

1. Describe the pathophysiology of glaucoma.
2. Identify clinical manifestations related to glaucoma.
3. Describe appropriate pharmacologic treatment of glaucoma.
4. Administer eyedrops safely and accurately.
5. Evaluate a patient's ability to correctly administer prescribed ophthalmic medication.

In this lesson you will learn the essentials of caring for a patient diagnosed with glaucoma. You will explore the patient's history, evaluate presenting symptoms and treatment, administer prescribed medications, and develop an individualized discharge teaching plan. Clarence Hughes is a 73-year-old male admitted for an elective left knee arthroplasty.

Exercise 1

 Clinical Preparation: Writing Activity

15 minutes

1. Briefly describe the general pathophysiology of glaucoma.

Copyright © 2007 by Mosby, Inc., an affiliate of Elsevier Inc. All rights reserved.

2. Compare and contrast the three different types of glaucoma by completing the following table.

Type of Glaucoma	Etiology	Pathophysiology	Clinical Manifestations
Primary open-angle			
Primary angle-closure			
Secondary			

3. Identify and describe measures used to diagnose glaucoma.

Copyright © 2007 by Mosby, Inc., an affiliate of Elsevier Inc. All rights reserved.

Exercise 2

 CD-ROM Activity

 45 minutes

- Sign in to work at Pacific View Regional Hospital for Period of Care 3. (*Note:* If you are already in the virtual hospital from a previous exercise, click on **Leave the Floor** and then **Restart the Program** to get to the sign-in window.)
- From the Patient List, select Clarence Hughes (Room 404).
- Click on **Go to Nurses' Station**.
- Click on **Chart** and then **404**.
- Click on **History and Physical**.

1. What problem of the eye does Clarence Hughes have?

2. How would this be diagnosed?

3. What signs and symptoms do you think he had prior to diagnosis?

4. What clinical manifestation(s) should you now assess for related to this diagnosis?

5. The H&P does not identify the type of glaucoma Clarence Hughes has. Based on his history and information in the textbook, which type do you think he mostly likely has? Explain why you came to this conclusion.

Copyright © 2007 by Mosby, Inc., an affiliate of Elsevier Inc. All rights reserved.

- Click on **Return to Nurses' Station**.
- Click on **MAR** and then on tab **404**.

6. What medications are ordered for Clarence Hughes' glaucoma? Identify these medications, their classifications, and mechanisms of action below. (*Note:* You will complete the last column in question 7.)

Medication	Drug Classification	Mechanism of Action	Side Effects

7. For what side effects should you monitor Clarence Hughes related to these medications? Record your answer in the table above.

8. If you were to administer the prescribed antiglaucoma medication to Clarence Hughes, how would you correctly apply the eye drops? Explain the step-by-step procedure. (*Hint:* Consult the Drug Guide by clicking on the **Drug** icon in the lower left corner of your screen.)

9. What range of IOP would Clarence Hughes have had prior to beginning treatment for glaucoma? What would you expect his reading to be during treatment?

Copyright © 2007 by Mosby, Inc., an affiliate of Elsevier Inc. All rights reserved.

→ • Click on **Return to Nurses' Station**.
  • Click on **Chart** and then **404**.
  • Click on **Patient Education**.

10. What educational goals would you add for Clarence Hughes related to his glaucoma?

11. What teaching would you provide for this patient regarding his glaucoma?

12. Complete the following table by documenting teaching points you would review with Clarence Hughes regarding his glaucoma medications.

Medication	Teaching Points

13. What teaching methods would you use to teach medication administration to this patient?

Copyright © 2007 by Mosby, Inc., an affiliate of Elsevier Inc. All rights reserved.

14. How would you evaluate Clarence Hughes' understanding of correct medication application?

15. If Clarence Hughes' ophthalmic medications would fail to maintain IOP within normal limits, what other therapies might he expect to undergo? Briefly describe each procedure.

Copyright © 2007 by Mosby, Inc., an affiliate of Elsevier Inc. All rights reserved.

LESSON **12**

Emphysema and Pneumonia

 Reading Assignment: Nursing Management: Lower Respiratory Problems
(Chapter 28)
Nursing Management: Obstructive Pulmonary Diseases
(Chapter 29)

Patient: Patricia Newman, Room 406

Goal: Utilize the nursing process to competently care for patients with altered oxygenation
states.

Objectives:

1. Relate physical assessment findings with pathophysiological changes of the lower respiratory tract.
2. Prioritize nursing care for a patient with altered oxygenation.
3. Evaluate laboratory results relative to the diagnosis of pneumonia and emphysema.
4. Describe pharmacological interventions related to altered oxygenation states.
5. Identify appropriate nursing interventions for a patient admitted with pneumonia and emphysema.
6. Identify appropriate discharge teaching needs for a patient with altered oxygenation.

In this lesson you will learn the essentials of caring for a patient diagnosed with pneumonia and emphysema. You will explore the patient's history, evaluate presenting symptoms and treatment on admission, and assess the patient's progress throughout the hospital stay. Patricia Newman is a 61-year-old female admitted with pneumonia and a history of emphysema. Begin this lesson by reviewing the general concepts of emphysema and pneumonia as presented in your textbook.

Exercise 1

 Clinical Preparation: Writing Activity

20 minutes

1. What category of lung diseases does emphysema belong to?

Copyright © 2007 by Mosby, Inc., an affiliate of Elsevier Inc. All rights reserved.

2. Briefly describe the pathophysiology of emphysema.

3. Briefly describe the pathophysiology of pneumonia.

4. Identify factors that may increase a patient's risk for developing pneumonia?

Copyright © 2007 by Mosby, Inc., an affiliate of Elsevier Inc. All rights reserved.

Exercise 2

  CD-ROM Activity

45 minutes

- Sign in to work at Pacific View Regional Hospital for Period of Care 1. (*Note:* If you are already in the virtual hospital from a previous exercise, click on **Leave the Floor** and then **Restart the Program** to get to the sign-in window.)
- From the Patient List, select Patricia Newman (Room 406).
- Click on **Get Report**.

1. What questions would you ask the outgoing nurses to obtain needed information not identified in report?

2. Below, relate the clinical manifestations identified in the change-of-shift report to the patient's diagnosis of pneumonia.

Clinical Manifestations	Pathophysiologic Basis
Labored respirations	
Use of accessory muscles	
Productive cough with yellow sputum	
Coarse breath sounds	
Lung infiltrates	
Disturbed sleep patterns	
Tachycardia	
Fever	

Copyright © 2007 by Mosby, Inc., an affiliate of Elsevier Inc. All rights reserved.

→ • Click on **Go to Nurses' Station**.
- Click on **Chart** and then **406**.
- Click on **History and Physical**.

3. What risk factors for community-acquired pneumonia does Patricia Newman have?

→ • Click on **Return to Nurses' Station**.
- Click on **406** to enter Patricia Newman's room.
- Read the **Initial Observation**.

4. What would be your priority nursing assessment/intervention(s) based on your initial observations of this patient?

→ • Click on **Patient Care** and perform a focused assessment based on Patricia Newman's admitting diagnosis.

5. Record your findings below. How has Patricia Newman's condition changed since report?

Focused Assessment Area	Assessment Findings	Change in Assessment
Respiratory		
Cardiovascular		
Mental Status		

Copyright © 2007 by Mosby, Inc., an affiliate of Elsevier Inc. All rights reserved.

• Click on **Nurse-Client Interactions**.

• Select and view the video titiled **0730: Prioritizing Interventions**. (*Note:* Check the virtual clock to see whether enough time has elapsed. You can use the fast-forward feature to advance the time by 2-minute intervals if the video is not yet available. Then click on **Patient Care** and **Nurse-Client Interactions** to refresh the screen.)

6. Evaluate the nurse's actions based on the patient's current status. How does this nurse's action differ from your plan of care in question 4?

 7. What nursing interventions would be appropriate to improve Patricia Newman's airway clearance and breathing pattern? (*Hint:* See Nursing Care Plan 28-1 in your textbook.)

 • Click on **Chart** and then **406**.

• Click on **Laboratory Reports**.

8. Identify any abnormal lab results and describe how they correlate with Patricia Newman's diagnosis of pneumonia.

Copyright © 2007 by Mosby, Inc., an affiliate of Elsevier Inc. All rights reserved.

• Click on **Return to Room 406**.
  • Click on **MAR** and then on tab **406**.

  9. What is the desired therapeutic effect of ipratropium bromide? How could the nurse assess whether the desired effect was achieved?

  10. What is the desired therapeutic effect of cefotetan? How could the nurse assess whether the desired effect was achieved?

  11. What is the rationale for administration of IV fluids related to pneumonia?

 • Click on **Medication Room**.
  • Click on **MAR** to determine medications that Patricia Newman is ordered to receive at 0800 and any appropriate prn medications you may want to administer. (*Note:* You may click on **Review MAR** at any time to verify the correct medication order. Remember to look at the patient name on the MAR to make sure you have the correct patient's record—you must click on the correct room number within the MAR. Click on **Return to Medication Room** after reviewing the correct MAR.)
  • Click on **Unit Dosage**. When the close-up view appears, click on drawer **406**.
  • Select the medication(s) you plan to administer. After each medication you select, click **Put Medication on Tray**. When you are finished, click on **Close Drawer**.
  • Click on **View Medication Room**.
  • Click on **IV Storage**. From the close-up view, click on the drawer labeled **Large Volume**.
  • Select the medication(s) you plan to administer, put the medication(s) on the tray, and close the bin.
  • Click **View Medication Room**.
  • Click on **Preparation**. Select the correct medication to administer; click **Prepare** and **Next**.
  • Choose the correct patient to administer this medication to and click **Finish**.
  • Repeat the above two steps until all medications that you want to administer are prepared.
  • You can click **Review Your Medications** and then **Return to Medication Room** when ready. From the Medication Room, you can go directly to Patricia Newman's room by clicking on **406** at the bottom of the screen.

Copyright © 2007 by Mosby, Inc., an affiliate of Elsevier Inc. All rights reserved.

- Administer the medication utilizing the five rights of medication administration. After you have collected the appropriate assessment data and are ready for administration, click **Patient Care** and then **Medication Administration**. Verify that the correct patient and medication(s) appear in the left-hand window. Then click the down arrow next to Select. From the drop-down menu, select **Administer** and complete the Administration Wizard by providing any information requested. When the Wizard stops asking for information, click **Administer to Patient**. Specify **Yes** when asked whether this administration should be recorded in the MAR. Finally, click **Finish**.

Now let's see how you did!

- Click on **Leave the Floor** at the bottom of your screen.
- From the Floor Menu, select **Look at Your Preceptor's Evaluation**.
- Click on **Medication Scorecard**.

12. Note below whether or not you correctly administered the appropriate medications. If not, why do you think you were incorrect? According to Table C in this scorecard, what are the appropriate resources that should be used and important assessments that should be completed before administering these medications? Did you use these resources and perform these assessments correctly?

Exercise 3

 CD-ROM Activity

 40 minutes

- Sign in to work at Pacific View Regional Hospital for Period of Care 2. (*Note:* If you are already in the virtual hospital from a previous exercise, click on **Leave the Floor** and then **Restart the Program** to get to the sign-in window.)
- From the Patient List, select Patricia Newman (Room 406).
- Click on **Go to Nurses' Station**.
- Click on **Chart** and then **406**.
- Click on **History and Physical**.

1. How long has Patricia Newman been diagnosed with emphysema?

Copyright © 2007 by Mosby, Inc., an affiliate of Elsevier Inc. All rights reserved.

2. What clinical manifestations documented on the H&P can be attributed to emphysema?

3. What additional clinical manifestations might you expect to see in other patients with emphysema?

➡ • Click on **Diagnostic Reports**.

4. What findings on the CXR are consistent with the diagnosis of emphysema?

5. What is the relationship between the patient's admitting diagnosis (pneumonia) and her underlying chronic condition (emphysema)?

➡ • Click on **Physician's Orders**.

6. What is the order for oxygen?

Copyright © 2007 by Mosby, Inc., an affiliate of Elsevier Inc. All rights reserved.

7. What is the rationale for this oxygen order as opposed to the usual goal of greater than 90% to 93% oxygen saturation? Is this appropriate? Why or why not? (*Hint:* See page 643 in your textbook.)

• Click on **Patient Education**.

8. What is educational goal 3 for Patricia Newman?

 9. Explain the rationale for using this technique. How would you teach the patient to achieve goal 3? (*Hint:* See page 646 in your textbook.)

10. What is educational goal 4 for Patricia Newman?

Copyright © 2007 by Mosby, Inc., an affiliate of Elsevier Inc. All rights reserved.

11. What do you think her special dietary needs are? Give a rationale for your answer.

12. What is educational goal 6 for Patricia Newman?

13. Explain the rationale for using this technique. How would you teach this patient to cough effectively? (*Hint:* See Table 29-25 on page 646 of your textbook.)

14. Since Patricia Newman's emphysema puts her at high risk for pulmonary infections, what would you teach her to do to help prevent further episodes of pneumonia? (*Hint:* See Health Promotion on pages 567-568, Ambulatory and Home Care on page 569, and Nursing Care Plan 29-2 on page 651 in your textbook.)

Copyright © 2007 by Mosby, Inc., an affiliate of Elsevier Inc. All rights reserved.

• Click on **Return to Nurses' Station**.
  • Click on **406** to go to Patricia Newman's room.
  • Click on **Patient Care** and then **Nurse-Client Interactions**.
  • Select and view the video titled **1100: Care Coordination**. (*Note:* Check the virtual clock to see whether enough time has elapsed. You can use the fast-forward feature to advance the time by 2-minute intervals if the video is not yet available. Then click on **Patient Care** and **Nurse-Client Interactions** to refresh the screen.)

15. What disciplines are involved in planning and providing care for Patricia Newman? List these in the left column below. In the right column, explain the role of each person in helping meet the patient's health care needs.

Involved Disciplines	Role in Patricia Newman's Health Care

Copyright © 2007 by Mosby, Inc., an affiliate of Elsevier Inc. All rights reserved.

LESSON 13

Asthma

👓 **Reading Assignment:** Nursing Assessment: Respiratory System (Chapter 26)
Nursing Management: Obstructive Pulmonary Diseases
(Chapter 29)

Patient: Jacquline Catanazaro, Room 402

Goal: Utilize the nursing process to competently care for patients with asthma.

Objectives:

1. Identify clinical manifestations of an acute asthmatic exacerbation.
2. Evaluate diagnostic tests as they relate to a patient's oxygenation status.
3. Describe medications used to treat asthma, including mechanism of action and therapeutic effects.
4. Prioritize nursing care for a patient with an acute exacerbation of asthma.
5. Formulate an appropriate patient education plan regarding home asthma management for a patient with identified barriers to learning.

In this lesson you will learn the essentials of caring for a patient diagnosed with asthma. You will explore the patient's history, evaluate presenting symptoms and treatment on admission, and follow the patient's progress throughout the hospital stay. Jacquline Catanazaro is a 45-year-old female admitted with increasing respiratory distress. Begin this lesson by reviewing the general concepts of asthma as presented in your textbook.

Copyright © 2007 by Mosby, Inc., an affiliate of Elsevier Inc. All rights reserved.

Exercise 1

Clinical Preparation: Writing Activity

30 minutes

1. Briefly describe the pathophysiology of asthma.

2. Compare and contrast the four classifications of asthma in the table below.

Classification of Asthma	Clinical Features
Step 1: Mild intermittent	
Step 2: Mild persistent	
Step 3: Moderate persistent	
Step 4: Severe persistent	

Copyright © 2007 by Mosby, Inc., an affiliate of Elsevier Inc. All rights reserved.

3. Define the following pulmonary function test measurements.

   a. Forced vital capacity (FVC)

   b. Forced expiratory volume in the first second (FEV_1)

   c. Peak expiratory flow rate (PEFR)

Exercise 2

 CD-ROM Activity

 40 minutes

- Sign in to work at Pacific View Regional Hospital for Period of Care 1. (*Note:* If you are already in the virtual hospital from a previous exercise, click on **Leave the Floor** and then **Restart the Program** to get to the sign-in window.)
- From the Patient List, select Jacquline Catanazaro (Room 402).
- Click on **Go to Nurses' Station**.
- Click on **Chart** and then **402**.
- Click on **History and Physical**.

1. What medical problems does Jacquline Catanazaro have?

Copyright © 2007 by Mosby, Inc., an affiliate of Elsevier Inc. All rights reserved.

2. What pathologic triggers can lead to an exacerbation of asthma?

3. Does Jacquline Catanazaro's history identify any of these triggers?

4. What other factor(s) might be contributing to her asthma exacerbations?

5. Based on her history and home medication regimen, what step of asthma management do you think she is normally at (excluding this admission for an exacerbation)? Explain.

→ • Click on **Emergency Department**.

6. What were Jacquline Catanazaro's presenting symptoms?

Copyright © 2007 by Mosby, Inc., an affiliate of Elsevier Inc. All rights reserved.

7. What diagnostic testing was ordered? Document and interpret the abnormal results below. (*Hint:* Review the Laboratory Reports and Diagnostic Reports sections of the chart to obtain these results.)

8. Read the ED physician's progress notes for 1400. What are the results of the patient's PEFR? How would you interpret these in light of her present condition? (*Hint:* Her predicted PEFR is >200 L/min.)

→ • Click on **Physician's Orders**.

9. What medical treatment is ordered in the ED? (*Hint:* See orders for Monday at 1005.)

10. How would you evaluate the patient's response to medical treatment?

Copyright © 2007 by Mosby, Inc., an affiliate of Elsevier Inc. All rights reserved.

11. What medications were ordered on Monday at 1600? What is the mechanism of action for each of these medications? (*Hint:* Click on **Return to Nurses' Station**; then click on the **Drug** icon in the lower left corner of your screen.)

12. Do these medications need to be adminstered in any specific order? Provide a rationale.

13. What new medications are ordered on Tuesday at 0800? Give a rationale for these orders. Why is the prednisone ordered to be decreased by 5 mg every day?

Copyright © 2007 by Mosby, Inc., an affiliate of Elsevier Inc. All rights reserved.

Exercise 3

 CD-ROM Activity

 30 minutes

- Sign in to work at Pacific View Regional Hospital for Period of Care 1. (*Note:* If you are already in the virtual hospital from a previous exercise, click on **Leave the Floor** and then **Restart the Program** to get to the sign-in window.)
- From the Patient List, select Jacquline Catanazaro (Room 402).
- Click on **Go to Nurses' Station**.
- Click on **402**.
- Inside the patient's room, read the **Initial Observations**.

1. Describe your initial observations when you enter Jacquline Catanazaro's room.

- Click on **Take Vital Signs**.

2. Record the patient's vital signs below.

3. Are there any clinical alerts for Jacquline Catanazaro? If so, describe below.

4. How would you prioritize your care for her at this point?

- Click on **Patient Care**.

Copyright © 2007 by Mosby, Inc., an affiliate of Elsevier Inc. All rights reserved.

5. Perform a focused assessment on three priority areas, based on Jacquline Catanazaro's present status. Record your findings in the right column.

Focused Areas of Assessment	Jacquline Catanazaro's Assessment Findings

 • Click on **Chart** and then **402**.
• Click on **Physician's Orders**.

6. What new orders did the physician write on Monday at 0730?

 • Click on **Return to Room 402**.
• Click on **Patient Care** and then **Nurse-Client Interactions**.
• Select and view the video titled **0730: Intervention—Anxiety**. (*Note:* Check the virtual clock to see whether enough time has elapsed. You can use the fast-forward feature to advance the time by 2-minute intervals if the video is not yet available. Then click on **Patient Care** and **Nurse-Client Interactions** to refresh the screen.)

Copyright © 2007 by Mosby, Inc., an affiliate of Elsevier Inc. All rights reserved.

7. How does this nurse prioritize her actions? What reasons can you give for this?

→ • Click on **Clinical Alerts**.

8. Look at the 0800 clinical alert. Interpret this alert below.

→ • Click on **Chart** and then **402**.
  • Click on **Physician's Notes**.

9. Read the notes for Wednesday at 0800. How does the physician evaluate the patient's condition at this point?

→ • Click on **Physician's Orders**. Find the orders for 0800 on Wednesday.

10. Record the orders below and provide a rationale for each.

New Orders	Rationale/Expected Therapeutic Response

 11. What noninvasive method might be useful to determine the effectiveness of treatment for Jacquline Catanazaro's acute asthma? Explain. (*Hint:* See page 615 in your textbook.)

Copyright © 2007 by Mosby, Inc., an affiliate of Elsevier Inc. All rights reserved.

Exercise 4

 CD-ROM Activity

 45 minutes

- Sign in to work at Pacific View Regional Hospital for Period of Care 2. (*Note:* If you are already in the virtual hospital from a previous exercise, click on **Leave the Floor** and then **Restart the Program** to get to the sign-in window.)
- From the Patient List, select Jacquline Catanazaro (Room 402).
- Click on **Get Report**.

1. Briefly summarize the activity for Jacquline Catanazaro over the last four hours.

- Click on **Go to Nurses' Station**.
- Click on **402** to go to the patient's room.

2. What is your initial observation of Jacquline Catanazaro for this time period?

3. Are there any clinical alerts?

- Click on **Take Vital Signs**.

4. Record Jacquline Catanazaro's current vital signs below. How do these results compare with those you obtained during Period of Care 1? (*Hint:* See Exercise 3, question 2 of this lesson.)

Copyright © 2007 by Mosby, Inc., an affiliate of Elsevier Inc. All rights reserved.

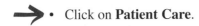 • Click on **Patient Care**.

5. Perform a focused assessment on Jacquline Catanazaro. Record your findings below. Then compare the findings with your assessment during Period of Care 1 and interpret your results. (*Hint:* See Exercise 3, question 5.)

Focused Areas of Assessment	Current Findings	Comparison with 0800 Findings—Interpretation of Results

 • Click on **Nurse-Client Interactions**.
• Select and view the video titled **1115: Assessment—Readiness to Learn**. (*Note:* Check the virtual clock to see whether enough time has elapsed. You can use the fast-forward feature to advance the time by 2-minute intervals if the video is not yet available. Then click on **Patient Care** and **Nurse-Client Interactions** to refresh the screen.)

6. Describe the nurse's actions. Are they appropriate? Explain.

7. What barriers to learning might be present for Jacquline Catanazaro?

Copyright © 2007 by Mosby, Inc., an affiliate of Elsevier Inc. All rights reserved.

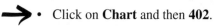 • Click on **Chart** and then **402**.
 • Click on **Patient Education**.

8. What are the educational goals for Jacquline Catanazaro?

9. What other asthma management needs would you teach this patient? (*Hint:* See Health Promotion discussion on pages 624-629 in your textbook.)

10. Describe the differences in outcomes met for Jacquline Catanazaro and her sister.

Copyright © 2007 by Mosby, Inc., an affiliate of Elsevier Inc. All rights reserved.

11. The patient is scheduled for discharge tomorrow. Do you have any concerns? What would be your most appropriate action?

 • Click on **Return to Room 402**.
- Click on **Leave the Floor**.
- Click on **Restart the Program**.
- Sign in to work at Pacific View Regional Hospital for Period of Care 3.
- From the Patient List, select Jacquline Catanazaro (Room 402).
- Click on **Go to Nurses' Station**.
- Click on **402**.
- Click on **Patient Care** and then **Nurse-Client Interactions**.
- Select and view the video titled **1500: Intervention—Patient Teaching**. (*Note:* Check the virtual clock to see whether enough time has elapsed. You can use the fast-forward feature to advance the time by 2-minute intervals if the video is not yet available. Then click on **Patient Care** and **Nurse-Client Interactions** to refresh the screen.)

12. What equipment is the nurse teaching Jacquline Catanazaro about?

 13. Describe proper use of the peak flow meter for this patient. (*Hint:* See Table 29-14 in your textbook.)

Copyright © 2007 by Mosby, Inc., an affiliate of Elsevier Inc. All rights reserved.

14. Describe the proper technique for use of a metered-dose inhaler (MDI). (*Hint:* See Figure 29-5 in your textbook.)

Copyright © 2007 by Mosby, Inc., an affiliate of Elsevier Inc. All rights reserved.

LESSON 14

Blood Component Therapy

🕮 **Reading Assignment:** Nursing Assessment: Hematologic System (Chapter 30, pages 672-674)

Nursing Management: Hematologic Problems (Chapter 31)

Patient: Piya Jordan, Room 403

Goal: Utilize the nursing process to competently care for patients receiving various blood products.

Objectives:

1. Describe the ABO and Rh antigen systems.
2. Identify the correct type of blood to administer to a specific patient.
3. Describe appropriate nursing responsibilities related to blood product administration.
4. Evaluate vital sign assessments related to potential blood transfusion reactions.
5. Describe appropriate assessment parameters when monitoring for various types of transfusion reactions.

In this lesson you will learn the essentials of caring for a patient receiving blood and blood product transfusions. You will describe pretransfusion responsibilities, identify administration specifics, and evaluate the patient during and after each transfusion. Piya Jordan is a 68-year-old female admitted with nausea, vomiting, and abdominal pain.

Copyright © 2007 by Mosby, Inc., an affiliate of Elsevier Inc. All rights reserved.

Exercise 1

Clinical Preparation: Writing Activity

10 minutes

1. Describe the ABO antigen system.

2. Describe the Rh antigen system.

3. Complete the table below to identify which types of blood are compatible with each other. (*Hint:* Use textbook Table 30-10, reading the recipient blood type at the top of the column and looking down the column to see what donor type each recipient can receive.)

Patient's Blood Type	Blood Types Patient Can Receive
A+	
A–	
B+	
B–	
O+	
O–	
AB+	
AB–	

Copyright © 2007 by Mosby, Inc., an affiliate of Elsevier Inc. All rights reserved.

Exercise 2

 CD-ROM Activity

 30 minutes

- Sign in to work at Pacific View Regional Hospital for Period of Care 1. (*Note:* If you are already in the virtual hospital from a previous exercise, click on **Leave the Floor** and then **Restart the Program** to get to the sign-in window.)
- From the Patient List, select Piya Jordan (Room 403).
- Click on **Go to Nurses' Station**.
- Click on **Chart** and then **403**.
- Click on **Laboratory Reports**.

1. Document the results of Piya Jordan's hematology results below.

	Monday 2200	Tuesday 0630	Wednesday 0630
Hemoglobin			
Hematocrit			

2. Why do you think her H&H is lower on Wednesday? (*Hint:* Check the Physican's Notes in the chart.)

 - Click on **Physician's Orders**.

3. What was ordered to correct this? Is this appropriate related to Piya Jordan's level of hemoglobin? Explain why or why not.

Copyright © 2007 by Mosby, Inc., an affiliate of Elsevier Inc. All rights reserved.

• Click on **Return to Nurses' Station**.
- Click on **403** to enter Piya Jordan's room.
- Click on **Patient Care** and then **Nurse-Client Interactions**.
- Select and view the video titled **0735: Pain—Adverse Drug Event**. (*Note:* Check the virtual clock to see whether enough time has elapsed. You can use the fast-forward feature to advance the time by 2-minute intervals if the video is not yet available. Then click on **Patient Care** and **Nurse-Client Interactions** to refresh the screen.)

4. What does the nurse state she will do to prepare the patient for a blood transfusion?

5. What gauge IV would you insert for the blood transfusion?

6. What other pretransfusion responsibilities would you complete? Have these been completed? (*Hint:* Check the patient's chart.)

 • Click on **Chart** and then **403**.
- Click on **Laboratory Reports**.

7. What day and time was the cross-match completed? What is the purpose of this lab test?

8. Explain how you would prepare the blood set-up prior to administration.

Copyright © 2007 by Mosby, Inc., an affiliate of Elsevier Inc. All rights reserved.

Exercise 3

  CD-ROM Activity

30 minutes

- Sign in to work at Pacific View Regional Hospital for Period of Care 2. (*Note:* If you are already in the virtual hospital from a previous exercise, click on **Leave the Floor** and then **Restart the Program** to get to the sign-in window.)
- From the Patient List, select Piya Jordan (Room 403).
- Click on **Go to Nurses' Station** and then **403** to enter Piya Jordan's room.
- Click on **Patient Care** and then **Nurse-Client Interactions**.
- Select and view the video titled **1115: Interventions—Nausea and Blood**. (*Note:* Check the virtual clock to see whether enough time has elapsed. You can use the fast-forward feature to advance the time by 2-minute intervals if the video is not yet available. Then click on **Patient Care** and **Nurse-Client Interactions** to refresh the screen.)

1. Piya Jordan's daughter verbalizes concern regarding the safety of blood transfusions. How did the nurse respond to this?

2. Describe how you would explain the safety of blood transfusions.

3. During the video, the nurse states that the blood has just arrived. How soon should the nurse begin the transfusion?

 - Click on **Chart** and then **403**.
- Click on **Laboratory Reports**.

4. What is Piya Jordan's blood type?

Copyright © 2007 by Mosby, Inc., an affiliate of Elsevier Inc. All rights reserved.

5. What type(s) of blood may she receive safely?

6. What baseline assessment is necessary prior to beginning the blood transfusion?

7. Describe the nurse's responsibilities during the initiation of this transfusion.

8. How fast would you transfuse this unit of blood? Give your rationale.

9. What assessments should be completed on Piya Jordan during the transfusion?

10. What would you document regarding this blood transfusion?

Copyright © 2007 by Mosby, Inc., an affiliate of Elsevier Inc. All rights reserved.

Exercise 4

CD-ROM Activity

🕐 40 minutes

- Sign in to work at Pacific View Regional Hospital for Period of Care 4. (*Note:* If you are already in the virtual hospital from a previous exercise, click on **Leave the Floor** and then **Restart the Program** to get to the sign-in window.)
- Click on **EPR** and then **Login**. (*Remember:* You are not able to visit patients or administer medications during Period of Care 4. You are able to review patients' records only.)
- Select **403** as the patient and **Vital Signs** as the category.

1. Below, document Piya Jordan's vital signs as recorded in the EPR after each of the two units of blood.

Time	Temp	Pulse	BP	Resp
1130				
1145				
1200				
1215				
1315				
1400				
1415				
1430				
1445				
1500				
1515				
1530				

2. According to the vital signs you recorded in question 1, did Piya Jordan have any adverse reactions to the blood transfusions? Explain.

Copyright © 2007 by Mosby, Inc., an affiliate of Elsevier Inc. All rights reserved.

3. What type of symptoms would you expect to see if she had a hemolytic transfusion reaction?

4. How would these symptoms differ if she had an allergic transfusion reaction?

5. How can you determine that Piya Jordan did not have a febrile reaction if she was febrile at the beginning of the transfusion?

6. If Piya Jordan would have demonstrated clinical manifestations indicative of a blood transfusion reaction, what would be the appropriate nursing interventions?

7. What was her total intake and output over the last 24 hours (i.e., Tuesday at 1500 through Wednesday at 1500)?

→ • Click on **Exit EPR**.
 • Click on **MAR** and then on tab **403**.

Copyright © 2007 by Mosby, Inc., an affiliate of Elsevier Inc. All rights reserved.

8. Over what period of time was the first unit of RBC infused? Was this appropriate? Explain.

9. What signs or symptoms would you expect to see if Piya Jordan was suffering from circulatory overload?

→ • Click on **Return to Nurses' Station**.
   • Click on **Chart** and then **403**.
   • Click on **Expired MARs**.

10. What other blood product has she received this admission? (*Hint:* Check Tuesday's MAR.)

11. How does this product differ from RBCs? Why was it given to Piya Jordan? (*Hint:* Check the History and Physical to determine reason for giving it.)

Copyright © 2007 by Mosby, Inc., an affiliate of Elsevier Inc. All rights reserved.

12. How does administration of FFP differ from administration of RBCs? (*Hint:* See Table 31-32 in your textbook.)

Copyright © 2007 by Mosby, Inc., an affiliate of Elsevier Inc. All rights reserved.

LESSON 15 ——————————————————————————

Hypertension

———————————————————————————————————————

👓 **Reading Assignment:** Nursing Management: Hypertension (Chapter 33)

Patients: Harry George, Room 401
　　　　　　Patricia Newman, Room 406

Goal: Utilize the nursing process to competently care for patients with hypertension.

Objectives:

1. Describe the classifications of blood pressure.
2. Identify the presence of risk factors for hypertension in assigned patients.
3. Discuss pharmacologic therapies available to treat hypertension.
4. Perform appropriate assessments prior to administering pharmacologic therapy for hypertension.
5. Develop an extensive educational plan for patients with hypertension.

In this lesson you will learn the essentials of caring for patients with hypertension. You will explore each patient's history, evaluate presenting symptoms and treatment, identify blood pressure classification, provide appropriate nursing interventions, and plan an appropriate patient educational plan related to the hypertension. Patricia Newman is a 61-year-old female admitted with pneumonia and a history of emphysema. Harry George is a 54-year-old male admitted with infection and swelling of the left foot.

Copyright © 2007 by Mosby, Inc., an affiliate of Elsevier Inc. All rights reserved.

Exercise 1

Clinical Preparation: Writing Activity

20 minutes

1. Identify and describe the classifications of blood pressure as presented in your textbook.

2. Identify and describe four physiologic controls of blood pressure.

   a.

   b.

Copyright © 2007 by Mosby, Inc., an affiliate of Elsevier Inc. All rights reserved.

c.

d.

3. Define the following terms.

a. Primary (essential) hypertension

b. Secondary hypertension

Copyright © 2007 by Mosby, Inc., an affiliate of Elsevier Inc. All rights reserved.

4. List the risk factors for primary (essential) hypertension.

    a.

    b.

    c.

    d.

    e.

    f.

    g.

    h.

    i.

    j.

    k.

    l.

    m.

Exercise 2

 CD-ROM Activity

 45 minutes

- Sign in to work at Pacific View Regional Hospital for Period of Care 1. (*Note:* If you are already in the virtual hospital from a previous exercise, click on **Leave the Floor** and then **Restart the Program** to get to the sign-in window.)
- From the Patient List, select Patricia Newman (Room 406).
- Click on **Go to Nurses' Station**.
- Click on **Chart** and then **406**.
- Click on **History and Physical**.

1. How long has Patricia Newman been diagnosed with hypertension?

 • Click on **Nursing Admission**.

2. What risk factors for hypertension does she have?

 • Click on **Physician's Orders**.

Copyright © 2007 by Mosby, Inc., an affiliate of Elsevier Inc. All rights reserved.

3. In the left column below, list all medications ordered to treat Patricia Newman's hypertension. For each medication, identify the drug classification and mechanism of action. (*Note:* You will complete the table in questions 4 and 5.)

Medication	Drug Classification	Mechanism of Action	Nursing Assessments	Side Effects

Copyright © 2007 by Mosby, Inc., an affiliate of Elsevier Inc. All rights reserved.

→ • Click on **Return to Nurses' Station**.
  • Click on the **Drug Guide** on the counter.

4. What nursing assessments are important before administering each of the medications you listed in question 3? Record your answers in the fourth column of the table.

5. For what side effects will the nurse need to monitor the patient? Record these in the last column of the table following question 3. (*Hint:* You may also use your textbook as a resource.)

→ • Click on **Return to Nurses' Station**.
  • Click **EPR** and then **Login**.
  • Select **406** as the patient and **Vital Signs** as the category.

6. What are Patricia Newman's documented blood pressure measurements since admission?

7. Is her prescribed antihypertensive medication currently effective?

8. In what classification of blood pressure would you place Patricia Newman based on her most current readings? Explain.

→ • Click on **Exit EPR**.
  • Click on **406** to go to the patient's room.
  • Click on **Patient Care** and then **Nurse-Client Interactions**.
  • Select and view the video titled **0740: Evaluation—Response to Care**. (*Note:* Check the virtual clock to see whether enough time has elapsed. You can use the fast-forward feature to advance the time by 2-minute intervals if the video is not yet available. Then click on **Patient Care** and **Nurse-Client Interactions** to refresh the screen.)

9. What might be contributing to Patricia Newman's currently elevated blood pressure?

Copyright © 2007 by Mosby, Inc., an affiliate of Elsevier Inc. All rights reserved.

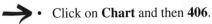 • Click on **Chart** and then **406**.
- Click on **History and Physical**.

10. What indicates that this patient is in need of further teaching regarding hypertension?

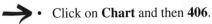 • Click on **Patient Education**.

11. What additional educational goals would be appropriate for Patricia Newman?

12. Develop a comprehensive teaching plan for this patient regarding nonpharmacological measures to treat hypertension.

Copyright © 2007 by Mosby, Inc., an affiliate of Elsevier Inc. All rights reserved.

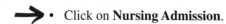 • Click on **Nursing Admission**.

13. Was Patricia Newman following any of the interventions you identified in question 12 to reduce her blood pressure at home? Explain.

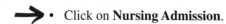 • Click on **Physician's Orders**.

14. Identify any of the interventions addressed in question 12 that were ordered for this patient during this hospital stay.

15. As the nurse caring for Patricia Newman, what do you think would be your professional responsibility related to your findings for questions 13 and 14?

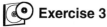 **Exercise 3**

 CD-ROM Activity

40 minutes

- Sign in to work at Pacific View Regional Hospital for Period of Care 1. (*Note:* If you are already in the virtual hospital from a previous exercise, click on **Leave the Floor** and then **Restart the Program** to get to the sign-in window.)
- From the Patient List, select Harry George (Room 401).
- Click on **Go to Nurses' Station**.
- Click on **EPR** and then **Login**.
- Select **401** as the patient and **Vital Signs** as the category.

Copyright © 2007 by Mosby, Inc., an affiliate of Elsevier Inc. All rights reserved.

1. Document Harry George's blood pressure results below.

	Tues 0305	Tues 0705	Tues 1105	Tues 1505	Tues 1905	Tues 2305	Wed 0305	Wed 0705
Blood pressure								

 • Click on **Exit EPR**.
- Click on **Chart** and then **401**.
- Click on **History and Physical**.

2. Does Harry George have a history of hypertension?

3. Does he have any risk factors for hypertension? If yes, please identify.

4. Based on the blood pressure recordings in question 1, in what classification would you put Harry George's blood pressure?

5. For what potential complications should you assess Harry George related to untreated hypertension?

 • Click on **Physician's Orders**.

Copyright © 2007 by Mosby, Inc., an affiliate of Elsevier Inc. All rights reserved.

6. Several diagnostic tests were ordered by the physician. Although these tests may have been ordered for various purposes, they may specifically help to identify target organ disease. In the middle column below, indicate how each test might be helpful. (*Hint:* You may refer to a laboratory/diagnostic reference manual for help. You will complete this table in questions 7 and 8.)

Diagnostic Test	How Test Might Help Identify Target Organ Disease	Harry George's Results
Chest x-ray		
BUN		
Creatinine		
Urinalysis		

➤ • Click on **Diagnostic Reports**.

7. Record the result of the chest x-ray in the third column of the table above and indicate whether the results suggest the presence of target organ disease.

➤ • Click on **Laboratory Reports**.

8. Find and record the lab results for BUN, creatinine, and urinalysis in the table above. Indicate what these results mean related to target organ disease.

Copyright © 2007 by Mosby, Inc., an affiliate of Elsevier Inc. All rights reserved.

9. In the table below, identify the various classifications of hypertensive medications that might be used to treat Harry George's elevated blood pressure. For each classification, briefly describe the mechanism of action.

Drug Classification	Mechanism of Action
a.	
b.	
c.	
d.	
e.	
f.	
g.	
h.	
i.	
j.	
k.	
l.	
m.	
n.	

Copyright © 2007 by Mosby, Inc., an affiliate of Elsevier Inc. All rights reserved.

10. What symptoms might Harry George display if his diastolic blood pressure dramatically increased above 140 mm Hg with a systolic blood pressure greater than 180 mm Hg?

11. What determines the seriousness of the patient's condition in hypertensive emergency?

12. Wht measurement will the health care team use to guide and evaluate therapy during a hypertensive emergency?

13. Describe the collaborative management of a patient with a hypertensive emergency.

Copyright © 2007 by Mosby, Inc., an affiliate of Elsevier Inc. All rights reserved.

Atrial Fibrillation

 Reading Assignment: Nursing Management: Dysrythmias (Chapter 36)

Patient: Piya Jordan, Room 403

Goal: Utilize the nursing process to competently care for patients with dysrhythmias.

Objectives:

1. Describe telemetry rhythm strip characteristics of atrial fibrillation.
2. Identify potential etiological causes of atrial fibrillation for an assigned patient.
3. Assess a patient for clinical manifestations of atrial fibrillation.
4. Develop a plan of care to monitor a patient for potential complications of atrial fibrillation.
5. Perform appropriate assessments prior to administering pharmacologic therapy for atrial fibrillation.
6. Accurately administer IV digoxin.
7. Discuss the use of anticoagulation therapy for a patient with atrial fibrillation.
8. Develop appropriate educational outcomes for patient with history of atrial fibrillation.

In this lesson you will learn the essentials of caring for a patient with a cardiac dysrhythmia. You will explore the patient's history, evaluate presenting symptoms and treatment, provide appropriate nursing interventions, and plan an appropriate patient educational outcome related to the dysrhythmia. Piya Jordan is a 68-year-old female admitted with nausea, vomiting, and abdominal pain.

Exercise 1

Clinical Preparation: Writing Activity

20 minutes

1. Describe the conduction pathway of a normal cardiac impulse.

Copyright © 2007 by Mosby, Inc., an affiliate of Elsevier Inc. All rights reserved.

2. Identify the cardiac event represented by each of the following waves and measured intervals.

   a. P wave

   b. QRS wave

   c. T wave

   d. PR interval

   e. QT interval

3. Define the following terms.

   a. Automaticity

   b. Contractility

   c. Conductivity

   d. Excitability

   e. Absolute refractory phase

Copyright © 2007 by Mosby, Inc., an affiliate of Elsevier Inc. All rights reserved.

4. List the ten steps recommended by your textbook for a systematic approach to assessing cardiac rhythms.

   a.

   b.

   c.

   d.

   e.

   f.

   g.

   h.

   i.

   j.

5. What three questions should be considered when evaluating a patient's cardiac rhythms?

   a.

   b.

   c.

Exercise 2

 CD-ROM Activity

 35 minutes

- Sign in to work at Pacific View Regional Hospital for Period of Care 1. (*Note:* If you are already in the virtual hospital from a previous exercise, click on **Leave the Floor** and then **Restart the Program** to get to the sign-in window.)
- From the Patient List, select Piya Jordan (Room 403).
- Click on **Go to Nurses' Station**.
- Click on **403** to enter Piya Jordan's room.

1. What information regarding cardiovascular status is obtained on initial observation of this patient?

Copyright © 2007 by Mosby, Inc., an affiliate of Elsevier Inc. All rights reserved.

2. What is telemetry monitoring?

3. What is atrial fibrillation?

4. Describe the rhythm strip you would expect to see on Piya Jordan's monitor.

5. How does normal sinus rhythm (NSR) differ from atrial fibrillation?

6. The nurse should monitor Piya Jordan for clinical manifestations of what physiologic deficit that might occur related to atrial fibrillation?

→ • Click on **Patient Care** and perform a general assessment of this patient.

Copyright © 2007 by Mosby, Inc., an affiliate of Elsevier Inc. All rights reserved.

7. Does Piya Jordan exhibit any symptoms of decreased cardiac output related to the atrial fibrillation? If so, describe the symptoms. If not, how would you explain that?

8. If the patient's heart rate increases, how might the atrial fibrillation affect her blood pressure? Describe underlying physiology. (*Hint:* Think about normal atrial-ventricular synchrony.)

 • Click on **Chart** and then **403**.
- Click on **Diagnostic Reports**.

9. Did Piya Jordan have a 12-lead ECG done? If yes, what was the rhythm? If not, do you think it should have been done? Why or why not?

10. For what specific complication related to atrial fibrillation is Piya Jordan at increased risk?

Copyright © 2007 by Mosby, Inc., an affiliate of Elsevier Inc. All rights reserved.

Exercise 3

 CD-ROM Activity

 45 minutes

- Sign in to work at Pacific View Regional Hospital for Period of Care 1. (*Note:* If you are already in the virtual hospital from a previous exercise, click on **Leave the Floor** and then **Restart the Program** to get to the sign-in window.)
- From the Patient List, select Piya Jordan (Room 403).
- Click on **Go to Nurses' Station**.
- Click on **MAR** and then select tab **403**.

1. What medication is prescribed to treat Piya Jordan's atrial fibrillation? Describe the pharmacodynamics of this medication as related to atrial fibrillation. (*Hint:* You may need to consult the Drug Guide.)

2. Why did the physician order a digoxin level when the patient first presented to the ED? (*Hint:* Review her presenting symptoms, as well as the Drug Guide.)

 • Click on **Return to Room 403**.
- Click on **Chart** and then **403**.
- Click on **Laboratory Reports**.

3. What was the digoxin level? Is this therapeutic or toxic?

Copyright © 2007 by Mosby, Inc., an affiliate of Elsevier Inc. All rights reserved.

4. For what other symptoms would you monitor Piya Jordan in relation to digoxin toxicity?

5. What was the patient's potassium level on admission to the ED?

6. How does this relate to possible digoxin toxicity?

➔ • Click on **History and Physical**.

7. What other medication was prescribed for Piya Jordan related to atrial fibrillation prior to this admission? Explain the rationale for this medication. (*Hint:* Think of potential serious complications of atrial fibrillation.)

➔ • Click on **Physician's Orders**.

8. What two items did the physician prescribe preoperatively to reverse Piya Jordan's anticoagulation? How would you know whether this was effective? Please explain.

Copyright © 2007 by Mosby, Inc., an affiliate of Elsevier Inc. All rights reserved.

9. What was ordered postoperatively to prevent clot formation?

→ • Click on **Nursing Admission**.

10. What knowledge (or lack of) does Piya Jordan verbalize regarding her history of atrial fibrillation? (*Hint:* Check the Health Promotion section.)

→ • Click on **Patient Education**.

11. What might you add to these outcomes based on your answer to question 10?

12. How would treatment for Piya Jordan differ if her atrial fibrillation was a new acute onset and the physician was trying to return her to a normal sinus rhythm rather than just control her heart rate?

13. What diagnostic procedure would you expect to be performed prior to DC cardioversion? Why?

Copyright © 2007 by Mosby, Inc., an affiliate of Elsevier Inc. All rights reserved.

14. What other treatment options may be used for patients with recurrent or sustained atrial fibrillation that is not responsive to medical management? Briefly explain the procedures.

- Click on **Return to Nurses' Station**.
- Click on **Medication Room**.
- Click on **MAR** to determine medications that Piya Jordan is ordered to receive at 0800. (*Note:* You may click on **Review MAR** at any time to verify correct medication order. Remember to look at the patient's name on the MAR to make sure you have the correct record—you must click on the correct room number within the MAR. Click on **Return to Medication Room** after reviewing the correct MAR.)
- Based on your care for Piya Jordan, access the various storage areas of the Medication Room to obtain the necessary medications you need to administer.
- For each area you access, first select the medication you plan to administer, then click **Put Medication on Tray**. When finished with a storage area, click on **Close Drawer**.
- Click **View Medication Room**.
- Click on **Preparation** and choose the correct medication to administer. Click **Prepare**.
- Click **Next** and choose the correct patient to administer this medication to. Click **Finish**.
- Repeat the above two steps until all medications that you want to administer are prepared.
- You can click **Review Your Medications** and then **Return to Medication Room** when you are ready. Once you are back in the Medication Room, you can go directly to Piya Jordan's room by clicking on **403** at the bottom of the screen.
- Administer the medication(s) utilizing the five rights of medication administration. After you have collected the appropriate assessment data and are ready for administration, click **Patient Care** and then **Medication Administration**. Verify that the correct patient and medication(s) appear in the left-hand window. Then click the down arrow next to Select. From the drop-down menu, select **Administer** and complete the Administration Wizard by providing any information requested. When the Wizard stops asking for information, click **Administer to Patient**. Specify **Yes** when asked whether this administration should be recorded in the MAR. Finally, click **Finish**.

15. Over how many minutes would you administer the IV digoxin?

16. What should you have assessed before administering digoxin to Piya Jordan today?

Copyright © 2007 by Mosby, Inc., an affiliate of Elsevier Inc. All rights reserved.

Now let's see how you did!

 • Click on **Leave the Floor** at the bottom of your screen.
- From the Floor Menu, select **Look at Your Preceptor's Evaluation**.
- Click on **Medication Scorecard**.

17. Note below whether or not you correctly administered the appropriate medication(s). If not, why do you think you were incorrect? According to Table C in this scorecard, what resources should be used and what important assessments should be completed before administering the medication(s)? Did you utilize these resources and perform these assessments correctly?

Copyright © 2007 by Mosby, Inc., an affiliate of Elsevier Inc. All rights reserved.

Exercise 3

 CD-ROM Activity

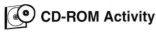 30 minutes

- Sign in to work at Pacific View Regional Hospital for Period of Care 3. (*Note:* If you are already in the virtual hospital from a previous exercise, click on **Leave the Floor** and then **Restart the Program** to get to the sign-in window.)
- From the Patient List, select Clarence Hughes (Room 404).
- Click on **Go to Nurses' Station**.
- Click on **Chart** and then **404**.
- Click on and review the **Laboratory Reports** and **Diagnostic Reports** sections of the chart.

1. Document the results of the diagnostic testing ordered for Clarence Hughes.

Diagnostic Test	Result

2. Based on the above results, what would you conclude to be the cause of Clarence Hughes' acute respiratory distress?

 3. What other diagnostic testing could the physician have ordered related to Clarence Hughes' pulmonary embolus? Explain the usefulness and/or significance of each test below and on the next page. (*Hint:* See page 599 in your textbook.) Spral CT, EKG, D-dimer

a.

b.

c.

Copyright © 2007 by Mosby, Inc., an affiliate of Elsevier Inc. All rights reserved.

$$\frac{10,000 \text{ units}}{1 mL} \times \frac{}{x mL}$$

d.

e.

f.

➤ • Click on **Physician's Orders**.

4. What orders were written to treat Clarence Hughes' pulmonary embolus?

heparin 80 units/kg stat bolus
bedrest
vital signs every 4 hrs

394
×80
00
180 kg/1 hr → 80 ×
→ 7,520
units

10,000
units/mL

5. What lab test will be used to titrate the heparin infusion? What are the normal values for this test?

1692
250
000 x

1692 ✳
60

6. What is the desired therapeutic level for this test? (*Hint:* Refer to the physician's orders.)

• Click on **Return to Nurses' Station**.
• Click on **MAR** and select tab **404**.

7. How many mL of heparin would you administer for the bolus dose?

.75 mls

18

Copyright © 2007 by Mosby, Inc., an affiliate of Elsevier Inc. All rights reserved.

8. If you were the nurse starting the heparin infusion, at what rate would you set the IV pump to infuse this medication?

- Click on **Return to Nurses' Station**.
- Click on **Chart** and then **404**.
- Click on **Laboratory Reports**.

9. What were the results of the PTT and INR at 1300 today? Why were these tests ordered prior to starting the heparin?

- Click on **Return to Nurses' Station**.
- Click on **404** to enter Clarence Hughes' room.
- Click on **Patient Care** and then **Nurse-Client Interactions**.
- Select and view the video titled **1510: Disease Management**. (*Note:* Check the virtual clock to see whether enough time has elapsed. You can use the fast-forward feature to advance the time by 2-minute intervals if the video is not yet available. Then click on **Patient Care** and **Nurse-Client Interactions** to refresh the screen.)

10. When Clarence Hughes' son asks the nurse whether the pulmonary embolism would delay his father's discharge, the nurse states that the heparin takes 2 days to stabilize. Does this mean that the patient will be discharged on heparin? If not, what medication will be used to minimize clot formation? Explain why the patient is not started on this medication rather than heparin.

Copyright © 2007 by Mosby, Inc., an affiliate of Elsevier Inc. All rights reserved.

11. What lab tests will be used to monitor the therapeutic effect of Coumadin? What is the therapeutic range for these tests? (*Hint:* You may need to use a diagnostic lab reference.)

12. For what possible complications would you monitor Clarence Hughes related to the pulmonary embolism?

— infarct his lungs
— shock → die

Exercise 4

 CD-ROM Activity

 30 minutes

- Sign in to work at Pacific View Regional Hospital for Period of Care 4. (*Note:* If you are already in the virtual hospital from a previous exercise, click on **Leave the Floor** and then **Restart the Program** to get to the sign-in window.)
- Click on **Chart** and then **404**. (*Remember:* You are not able to visit patients or administer medications during Period of Care 4. You are able to review patients' records only.)
- Click on **Laboratory Reports**.

1. What is the PTT result for 1900?

- Click on **Return to Nurses' Station**.
- Click on **MAR** and then on tab **404**.

2. What would you do now with the heparin infusion? Calculate the correct infusion rate and document below. (*Hint:* Refer to your answer for question 7 in Exercise 3.)

Copyright © 2007 by Mosby, Inc., an affiliate of Elsevier Inc. All rights reserved.

• Click on **Return to Nurses' Station**.

• Click on **Kardex** and choose tab **404**. Review the stated outcomes for Clarence Hughes.

3. Should other outcomes be added because of his pulmonary embolus? Give rationale.

4. If the heparin is not effective in treating Clarence Hughes and/or his condition worsens, what other pharmacologic treatment might be helpful? Explain.

 5. Describe bleeding precautions that must be followed while the patient is receiving heparin therapy. (*Hint:* See Table 38-13 in your textbook.)

Copyright © 2007 by Mosby, Inc., an affiliate of Elsevier Inc. All rights reserved.

6. If Clarence Hughes' condition deteriorates, what surgical treatment would be needed? Explain.

7. If the patient develops another pulmonary embolism, what further treatment might the physician consider to prevent the recurrence of PEs? Explain.

Copyright © 2007 by Mosby, Inc., an affiliate of Elsevier Inc. All rights reserved.

LESSON **18** ——————————————————————

Nutritional Problems

/∞ **Reading Assignment:** Nursing Management: Nutritional Problems (Chapter 40)
Nursing Management: Obesity (Chapter 41)

Patients: Harry George, Room 401
Jacquline Catanazaro, Room 402
Piya Jordan, Room 403

Goal: Utilize the nursing process to competently care for patients with nutritional disorders.

Objectives:

1. Identify patients at risk for malnutrition.
2. Perform a nutritional screening assessment on assigned patients.
3. Evaluate laboratory findings in relation to a patient's nutritional status.
4. Plan appropriate dietary interventions for a patient with malnutrition.
5. Identify a patient's risk factors related to obesity.
6. Formulate an appropriate patient education plan for an overweight patient.

In this lesson you will learn the essentials of caring for patients with nutritional disorders. You will explore each patient's history, perform a nutritional screening assessment, evaluate findings, and plan appropriate nursing interventions, including the patient's educational needs. Harry George is a 54-year-old male with a 4-year history of type 2 diabetes admitted with infection and swelling of his left foot. Piya Jordan is a 68-year-old female admitted with nausea and vomiting for several days following weeks of poor appetite and increasing weakness. Jacquline Catanazaro is a 45-year-old female admitted with an acute exacerbation of asthma.

Copyright © 2007 by Mosby, Inc., an affiliate of Elsevier Inc. All rights reserved.

Exercise 1

Clinical Preparation: Writing Activity

10 minutes

1. Describe the most recently revised Food Guide Pyramid. (*Hint:* Go to www.mypyramid.gov.)

2. Describe the recommended daily requirements for the following essential dietary components.

Carbohydrate

Protein

Fat

3. Describe the difference between complete and incomplete proteins. Give examples of each.

Copyright © 2007 by Mosby, Inc., an affiliate of Elsevier Inc. All rights reserved.

4. Identify and describe the three types of factors that influence obesity.

Exercise 2

 CD-Rom Activity

 40 minutes

- Sign in to work at Pacific View Regional Hospital for Period of Care 1. (*Note:* If you are already in the virtual hospital from a previous exercise, click on **Leave the Floor** and then **Restart the Program** to get to the sign-in window.)
- From the Patient List, select Harry George (Room 401) and Piya Jordan (Room 403).
- Click on **Go to Nurses' Station**.
- Click on **Chart** and then **401** for Harry George's chart.
- Click on **History and Physical**.

1. What risk factors for malnutrition are noted in Harry George's H&P?

- Click on **Return to Nurses' Station**.
- Click on **Chart** and then **403** for Piya Jordan's chart.
- Click on **History and Physical**.

2. What risk factors for malnutrition are noted in Piya Jordan's H&P?

Copyright © 2007 by Mosby, Inc., an affiliate of Elsevier Inc. All rights reserved.

- Click on **Return to Nurses' Station**.
- Click on **401** to enter Harry George's room.
- Click on **Patient Care**.

3. Although not every patient needs a complete nutritional assessment, it is essential to assess at-risk patients for symptoms of malnutrition. Referring to Table 40-9 in your textbook on page 956, assess Harry George for any of the identified findings associated with malnutrition. Obtain subjective information by reading his History and Physical, Nursing Admission form, and laboratory results. Gather the objective data by completing a physical assessment on the patient. Document your findings in column 2 below and on the next page. (*Note:* You will perform a similar assessment of Piya Jordan during Exercise 3 and record those findings in column 3.)

Screening Assessments Subjective Data	Harry George	Piya Jordan
Past health history		
Medications		
Surgery or other treatments		
Functional Health Patterns Health-Perception		
Nutritional-Metabolic		
Elimination		
Activity-Exercise		
Cognitive-Perceptual		
Role-Relationship		
Sexual-Reproductive		

Copyright © 2007 by Mosby, Inc., an affiliate of Elsevier Inc. All rights reserved.

Screening Assessments

Objective Data	Harry George	Piya Jordan
General		
Integumentary		
Eyes		
Respiratory		
Cardiovascular		
Gastrointestinal		
Neurologic		
Musculoskeletal		
Laboratory findings		

Copyright © 2007 by Mosby, Inc., an affiliate of Elsevier Inc. All rights reserved.

4. Calculate Harry George's body mass index (BMI) based on his current height and weight by using the following formula:

$$\frac{\text{Weight in pounds}}{\text{Height in inches} \times \text{Height in inches}} \times 703 = \text{BMI}$$

5. Evaluate the results of your findings in questions 3 and 4. What clinical manifestations of protein-calorie malnutrition does Harry George display?

6. What is Harry George's degree of protein depletion? (*Hint:* See Table 40-10 in your textbook.)

7. Is Harry George's protein-calorie malnutrition (PCM) primary or secondary? Explain how you came to your conclusion.

Exercise 3

 CD-Rom Activity

 40 minutes

- Sign in to work at Pacific View Regional Hospital for Period of Care 1. (*Note:* If you are already in the virtual hospital from a previous exercise, click on **Leave the Floor** and then **Restart the Program** to get to the sign-in window.)
- From the Patient List, select Harry George (Room 401) and Piya Jordan (Room 403).
- Click on **Go to Nurses' Station**.
- Click on **403** to enter Piya Jordan's room.
- Click on **Patient Care**.

Copyright © 2007 by Mosby, Inc., an affiliate of Elsevier Inc. All rights reserved.

1. Now perform the same nutritional screening assessment on Piya Jordan as you did for Harry George in the previous exercise. Referring to Table 40-9 in your textbook on page 956, assess the patient for any of the identified findings associated with malnutrition. Obtain subjective information by reading her History and Physical, Nursing Admission form, and Laboratory Reports. Acquire the objective data by completing a physical assessment. Documenting your findings in column 3 of the table on the previous two pages.

2. Calculate Piya Jordan's BMI based on her current height and weight by using the following formula:

$$\frac{\text{Weight in pounds}}{\text{Height in inches} \times \text{Height in inches}} \times 703 = \text{BMI}$$

3. Evaluate the results of your findings for questions 1 and 2. What clinical manifestations of protein-calorie malnutrition, if any, does Piya Jordan display?

4. What is Piya Jordan's degree of protein depletion? (*Hint:* See Table 40-10 in your textbook.)

5. Is Piya Jordan's protein-calorie malnutrition (PCM) primary or secondary? Explain how you came to your conclusion.

Copyright © 2007 by Mosby, Inc., an affiliate of Elsevier Inc. All rights reserved.

6. Compare and contrast your findings for Harry George and Piya Jordan. What are the similarities? What are the differences?

7. What other laboratory tests, not ordered for either of these patients, might be useful in evaluating their nutritional status?

8. Identify two nursing diagnoses related to Piya Jordan's and Harry George's malnourished status.

9. What type of diet or dietary supplements would you recommend for these two patients?

10. What additional nursing interventions would be appropriate to address these patients' nutritional needs?

Copyright © 2007 by Mosby, Inc., an affiliate of Elsevier Inc. All rights reserved.

Exercise 4

 CD-ROM Activity

30 minutes

- Sign in to work at Pacific View Regional Hospital for Period of Care 2. (*Note:* If you are already in the virtual hospital from a previous exercise, click on **Leave the Floor** and then **Restart the Program** to get to the sign-in window.)
- From the Patient List, select Jacquline Catanazaro (Room 402).
- Click on **Go to Nurses' Station**.
- Click on **Chart** and then **402**.
- Click on **Nursing Admission**.

1. Document Jacquline Catanazaro's current height and weight below.

2. Calculate her BMI using the following formula:

$$\frac{\text{Weight in pounds}}{\text{Height in inches} \times \text{Height in inches}} \times 703 = \text{BMI}$$

3. Is Jacquline Catanazaro's nutritional status underweight, normal, overweight, obese, or morbidly obese?

→ • Click on **History and Physical**.

4. What complication of obesity does this patient suffer from?

Copyright © 2007 by Mosby, Inc., an affiliate of Elsevier Inc. All rights reserved.

5. Identify other complications Jacquline Catanazaro may be at risk for related to the following categories.

Cardiovascular

Respiratory

Metabolic

Musculoskeletal

Liver/Gallbladder

Gastrointestinal

Genitourinary

Reproductive

Psychologic

Cancer

6. What measurement could be used to assess Jacquline Catanazaro's risk for cardiovascular complications? Explain the significance of this measurement.

Copyright © 2007 by Mosby, Inc., an affiliate of Elsevier Inc. All rights reserved.

7. What are the contributing factors for Jacquline Catanazaro's increased weight?

→ • Click on **Return to Nurses' Station**.
  • Click on **MAR** and then on tab **402**.

8. Do any of the medications ordered for Jacquline Catanazaro cause weight gain? If so, describe. (*Hint:* Consult the Drug Guide provided in the Nurses' Station.)

→ • Click on **Return to Nurses' Station**.
  • Click on **402** to enter the patient's room.
  • Click on **Patient Care** and then **Nurse-Client Interactions**.
  • Select and view the video titled **1140: Compliance—Medications**. (*Note:* Check the virtual clock to see whether enough time has elapsed. You can use the fast-forward feature to advance the time by 2-minute intervals if the video is not yet available. Then click on **Patient Care** and **Nurse-Client Interactions** to refresh the screen.)

9. What concern does the patient voice regarding her medications?

10. Evaluate the nurse's response. Was it appropriate? Accurate?

11. What else could the nurse have suggested to help this patient lose weight?

Copyright © 2007 by Mosby, Inc., an affiliate of Elsevier Inc. All rights reserved.

12. What medications might be used as adjuncts to a diet and exercise program for Jacquline Catanazaro?

13. Is Jacquline Catanazaro a candidate for bariatric surgery? Why or why not?

14. If this patient had been morbidly obese, what other treatment options might she have?

Copyright © 2007 by Mosby, Inc., an affiliate of Elsevier Inc. All rights reserved.

19

Intestinal Obstruction/ Colorectal Cancer

⌒◯⌒ **Reading Assignment:** Nursing Management: Lower Gastrointestinal Problems
(Chapter 43)

Patient: Piya Jordan, Room 403

Goal: Utilize the nursing process to competently care for patients with lower gastrointestinal problems.

Objectives:

1. Correlate a patient's history and clinical manifestations with a diagnosis of intestinal obstruction.
2. Evaluate laboratory and diagnostic test results of a patient admitted with a noninflammatory intestinal disorder.
3. Plan appropriate nursing interventions for a patient with a nasogastric tube.
4. Prioritize nursing care for a patient with an intestinal obstruction.
5. Provide appropriate psychosocial interventions for a patient and family diagnosed with colon cancer.
6. Formulate an appropriate patient education plan for a postoperative patient with colorectal cancer.

In this lesson you will learn the essentials of caring for a patient admitted with an intestinal obstruction and diagnosed with colorectal cancer. You will explore the patient's history, evaluate presenting symptoms and treatment, plan appropriate nursing interventions, and develop an individualized teaching plan. Piya Jordan is a 68-year-old female admitted with nausea and vomiting for several days following weeks of poor appetite and increasing weakness.

Copyright © 2007 by Mosby, Inc., an affiliate of Elsevier Inc. All rights reserved.

Exercise 1

Clinical Preparation: Writing Activity

20 minutes

1. Describe the pathophysiology of fluid and electrolyte imbalances associated with an intestinal obstruction.

2. Compare and contrast mechanical and nonmechanical intestinal obstructions.

   a. Mechanical obstruction

   b. Nonmechanical obstruction

3. How does the removal of polyps help to prevent colorectal cancer? (*Hint:* Describe the relationship between polyps and cancer development.)

Copyright © 2007 by Mosby, Inc., an affiliate of Elsevier Inc. All rights reserved.

4. Identify the four most common sites of metastasis for colorectal cancer.

Exercise 2

 CD-ROM Activity

 40 minutes

- Sign in to work at Pacific View Regional Hospital for Period of Care 1. (*Note:* If you are already in the virtual hospital from a previous exercise, click on **Leave the Floor** and then **Restart the Program** to get to the sign-in window.)
- From the Patient List, select Piya Jordan (Room 403).
- Click on **Go to Nurses' Station**.
- Click on **Chart** and then **403**.
- Click on **Emergency Department**.

1. What were Piya Jordan's presenting symptoms?

 - Click on **History and Physical**.

2. What history of symptoms is recorded?

 - Click on **Laboratory Reports**.

3. Document Piya Jordan's admission electrolyte results below and on the next page. Evaluate whether each of the results is normal, decreased, or increased. Offer your rationale for any abnormalities in the last column.

	Monday 2200	Decreased, Normal, or Increased?	Rationales for Abnormality
Sodium			

Copyright © 2007 by Mosby, Inc., an affiliate of Elsevier Inc. All rights reserved.

	Monday 2200	Decreased, Normal, or Increased?	Rationales for Abnormality
Potassium			
Chloride			
CO_2			
Creatinine			
BUN			
Amylase			

→ • Click on **Diagnostic Reports**.

4. What was the result of the patient's KUB? What do air-fluid levels indicate?

Copyright © 2007 by Mosby, Inc., an affiliate of Elsevier Inc. All rights reserved.

5. Why do you think a CT scan of the abdomen was ordered? What was the result?

6. What part of the bowel is the terminal ileum?

7. Was Piya Jordan's obstruction mechanical or nonmechanical? Explain.

8. For what priority problem related to intestinal obstruction should the nurse assess Piya Jordan?

9. If the patient had sought medical attention prior to the obstruction worsening, what other diagnostic testing might she have undergone? Explain what the test would show.

→ • Click on **History and Physical**.

Copyright © 2007 by Mosby, Inc., an affiliate of Elsevier Inc. All rights reserved.

10. Now that you know Piya Jordan has a colonic mass, let's look at those presenting symptoms again. Common clinical manifestations of colorectal cancer are listed below. Place an X next to each sign or symptom consistent with the patient's history and her physical examination findings on admission.

_____ a. Rectal bleeding

_____ b. Alternating constipation and diarrhea

_____ c. Anemia

_____ d. Fatigue

_____ e. Weakness

_____ f. Colicky abdominal pain

_____ g. Vague abdominal discomfort

_____ h. Sensation of incomplete emptying

_____ i. Change in stool caliber (narrow, ribbonlike)

_____ j. Weight loss

➤ • Click on **Physician's Orders**.

11. What IV fluid did the ED physician initially order? Why? (*Hint:* Look at Piya Jordan's vital signs in the Emergency Department record and relate them to fluid/electrolyte changes noted with intestinal obstruction.)

12. What else did the ED physician order to treat the intestinal obstruction? Explain the purpose of this intervention.

➤ • Click on **Return to Nurses' Station**.
  • Click on **403** to enter Piya Jordan's room.
  • Click on **Patient Care**.

Copyright © 2007 by Mosby, Inc., an affiliate of Elsevier Inc. All rights reserved.

13. Perform a focused abdominal assessment. Document your findings below.

14. Describe any additional assessments and/or interventions related to the NGT that you might do for Piya Jordan.

Exercise 3

 CD-ROM Activity

 45 minutes

- Sign in to work at Pacific View Regional Hospital for Period of Care 3. (*Note:* If you are already in the virtual hospital from a previous exercise, click on **Leave the Floor** and then **Restart the Program** to get to the sign-in window.)
- From the Patient List, select Piya Jordan (Room 403).
- Click on **Go to Nurses' Station**.
- Click on **Chart** and then **403**.
- Click on **History and Physical**.

1. Below is a list of risk factors for colorectal cancer. Place an X next to those that are documented in Piya Jordan's record.

_____   a. Age > 50 years

_____   b. Familial adematosis polyposis (colorectal polyps)

_____   c. Alcohol intake (4 or more drinks a week)

_____   d. Red meat intake (7 or more servings a week)

_____   e. Inflammatory bowel disease for 10 years or more

_____   f. Family history of colorectal cancer (first degree relative)

_____   g. Cigarette use

_____   h. Hereditary nonpolyposis colorectal cancer (HNPCC)

_____   i. Obesity (body mass index > 30 kg/m^2)

Copyright © 2007 by Mosby, Inc., an affiliate of Elsevier Inc. All rights reserved.

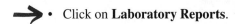 • Click on **Laboratory Reports**.

2. Below, document Piya Jordan's admission H&H. How would you explain the results?

	Monday 2200	Decreased, WNL, or Increased?	Rationale for Abnormality
Hemoglobin			
Hematocrit			

• Click on **Expired MARs**.

3. What was administered preoperatively to clean out Piya Jordan's bowel?

• Click on **Surgical Reports**.

4. Review the operative report. Name and describe the surgical procedure.

5. What is the most likely cell type for Piya Jordan's cancer?

6. How will the physician know what kind of cancer the tumor is?

Copyright © 2007 by Mosby, Inc., an affiliate of Elsevier Inc. All rights reserved.

7. Explain how you would classify Piya Jordan's tumor according to the following two staging systems.

    a. Duke's Classification System

    b. TNM Classification

→ • Click on **Laboratory Results**.

8. Why did the physician order an amylase, lipase, and LFTs? What do the results demonstrate?

→ • Click on **Return to Nurses' Station** and then **403**.
  • Click on **Patient Care** and then **Nurse-Client Interactions**.
  • Select and view the video titled **1500: Preventing Complications**. (*Note:* Check the virtual clock to see whether enough time has elapsed. You can use the fast-forward feature to advance the time by 2-minute intervals if the video is not yet available. Then click on **Patient Care** and **Nurse-Client Interactions** to refresh the screen.)

9. What nursing interventions are discussed during this brief video? Why are they appropriate for Piya Jordan?

→ • Click on **Patient Care** and then **Nurse-Client Interactions**.
  • Select and view the video titled **1540: Discharge Planning**. (*Note:* Check the virtual clock to see whether enough time has elapsed. You can use the fast-forward feature to advance the time by 2-minute intervals if the video is not yet available. Then click on **Patient Care** and **Nurse-Client Interactions** to refresh the screen.)

Copyright © 2007 by Mosby, Inc., an affiliate of Elsevier Inc. All rights reserved.

10. Piya Jordan's daughter seems to be overwhelmed by her mother's illness and needs. Describe psychosocial interventions that the nurse might plan to help Piya Jordan and her daughter.

11. What would you teach Piya Jordan's daughter regarding health promotion and prevention of colon cancer for herself?

Copyright © 2007 by Mosby, Inc., an affiliate of Elsevier Inc. All rights reserved.

LESSON **20**

Diabetes Mellitus, Part 1

Reading Assignment: Nursing Management: Diabetes Mellitus (Chapter 49)

Patient: Harry George, Room 401

Goal: Utilize the nursing process to competently care for patients with diabetes mellitus.

Objectives:

1. Describe the etiology of type 1 and type 2 diabetes mellitus.
2. Compare and contrast the characteristics of type 1 and type 2 diabetes.
3. Identify the relationship between diabetes and other disease processes.
4. Evaluate a patient's risk factors for diabetes.
5. Assess a patient for short- and long-term complications of diabetes.
6. Develop an appropriate plan of care for a patient with type 2 diabetes.

In this lesson you will learn the essentials of caring for a patient admitted with complications related to diabetes mellitus. You will explore the patient's history, evaluate presenting symptoms and treatment, plan appropriate nursing interventions, and develop an individualized teaching plan. Harry George is a 54-year-old male with a 4-year history of type 2 diabetes admitted with infection and swelling of his left foot.

Exercise 1

 Clinical Preparation: Writing Activity

 20 minutes

1. Briefly define and summarize the etiologic differences between type 1 and type 2 diabetes mellitus.

Type 1 diabetes mellitus

Copyright © 2007 by Mosby, Inc., an affiliate of Elsevier Inc. All rights reserved.

Type 2 diabetes mellitus

2. Compare and contrast the distinguishing characteristics of type 1 and type 2 diabetes mellitus (DM) by completing the table below.

Features	Type 1 DM	Type 2 DM
Age at onset		
Type of onset		
Primary defect		
Symptoms		
Endogenous insulin		
Prevalence		
Islet cell antibodies		
Environmental factors		
Ketosis		
Nutritional therapies		
Insulin		
Nutritional status		
Vascular and neurolgic complications		

Copyright © 2007 by Mosby, Inc., an affiliate of Elsevier Inc. All rights reserved.

Exercise 2

 CD-ROM Activity

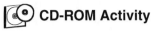 45 minutes

- Sign in to work at Pacific View Regional Hospital for Period of Care 1. (*Note:* If you are already in the virtual hospital from a previous exercise, click on **Leave the Floor** and then **Restart the Program** to get to the sign-in window.)
- From the Patient List, select Harry George (Room 401).
- Click on **Go to Nurses' Station**.
- Click on **Chart** and then **401**.
- Click on **History and Physical**.

1. What risk factors for diabetes are noted in Harry George's history?

2. Describe the history of this patient's present illness.

 3. What is the relationship between the infection in Harry George's foot and his diabetes mellitus? (*Hint:* Read about complications of the foot and lower extremity in your textbook.)

 - Click on **Laboratory Reports**.

4. What was Harry George's admitting blood glucose level?

5. What abnormalities in his urinalysis results can be attributed to the diabetes? Explain the relationship.

Copyright © 2007 by Mosby, Inc., an affiliate of Elsevier Inc. All rights reserved.

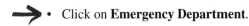 • Click on **Emergency Department**.

6. What factor in Harry George's recent history most likely contributed to his hyperglycemia? (*Hint:* Read the ED physician's notes for 1345.)

 • Click on **Nursing Admission**.

7. Listed below are clinical manifestations of diabetes mellitus identified in the textbook. In column 2, indicate (with Yes or No) whether each manifestation is usually present in type 2 diabetes. Then indicate (with Yes or No) whether Harry George displays each manifestation based on the nurse's initial assessment.

Clinical Manifestations	Present in Type 2 DM? (Yes or No)	Experienced by Harry George? (Yes or No)
Polyuria		
Polydipsia		
Polyphagia		
Visual changes		
Weakness/fatigue		
Weight loss		
Chronic complications		
Recurrent infections		
Prolonged wound healing		

8. To what extent does Harry George fit the typical picture of a patient with type 2 diabetes mellitus?

• Click on **Return to Nurses' Station** and then **401**.
• Click on **Patient Care** and then **Nurse-Client Interactions**.
• Select and view the video titled **0755: Disease Management**. (*Note:* Check the virtual clock to see whether enough time has elapsed. You can use the fast-forward feature to advance the time by 2-minute intervals if the video is not yet available. Then click on **Patient Care** and **Nurse-Client Interactions** to refresh the screen.)

Copyright © 2007 by Mosby, Inc., an affiliate of Elsevier Inc. All rights reserved.

9. What does Harry George tell the nurse about his appetite?

10. What diet has been ordered for the patient? (*Hint:* Review his chart.)

11. Describe the principles of this diet.

12. How might the patient's alcohol intake affect his blood glucose levels?

Exercise 3

CD-ROM Activity

40 minutes

- Sign in to work at Pacific View Regional Hospital for Period of Care 2. (*Note:* If you are already in the virtual hospital from a previous exercise, click on **Leave the Floor** and then **Restart the Program** to get to the sign-in window.)
- From the Patient List, select Harry George (Room 401).
- Click on **Go to Nurses' Station**.
- Click on **Chart** and then **401**.
- Click on **Physician's Orders**.

Copyright © 2007 by Mosby, Inc., an affiliate of Elsevier Inc. All rights reserved.

1. What test ordered can be used to determine Harry George's control of diabetes mellitus? Describe the purpose of this test.

2. What was the result of this test for Harry George? Evaluate and explain how well controlled his diabetes is based on these results.

3. What implication does the patient's issue of poor glycemic control have for his future?

→ • Click on **Return to Nurses' Station** and then **401** to enter Harry George's room.
   • Click on **Patient Care** and perform a head-to-toe assessment on the patient.

4. Below and on the next page, document any abnormal results from your assessment of Harry George.

Assessment Area	Assessment Results
Head & Neck	
Chest	
Back & Spine	

Copyright © 2007 by Mosby, Inc., an affiliate of Elsevier Inc. All rights reserved.

Assessment Area	Assessment Results
Upper Extremities	
Abdomen	
Pelvic	
Lower Extremities	

→ • Click on **EPR** and **Login**.
  • Select **401** as the patient and **Neurologic** as the category.

5. List any abnormal results from the neurologic assessment on Monday at 1835.

6. Describe the potential long-term complications for DM listed below and on the next page.

Macrovascular

Diabetic retinopathy

Copyright © 2007 by Mosby, Inc., an affiliate of Elsevier Inc. All rights reserved.

Neuropathy

Nephropathy

7. Does Harry George exhibit signs or symptoms that would alert you to the possibility of any of the long-term complications noted in question 6? If so, explain. (*Hint:* Consider your answers to questions 4 and 5 of this exercise, as well as question 5 in Exercise 2.)

8. What patient teaching would you plan to offer this patient to prevent further injury secondary to reduced sensation in his left foot? (*Hint:* See Table 49-22 in your textbook.)

9. Using correct NANDA format, state 3 nursing diagnoses related to Harry George's diabetes.

Copyright © 2007 by Mosby, Inc., an affiliate of Elsevier Inc. All rights reserved.

Diabetes Mellitus, Part 2

 Reading Assignment: Nursing Management: Diabetes Mellitus (Chapter 49)

Patient: Harry George, Room 401

Goal: Utilize the nursing process to competently administer medications prescribed to treat patients with diabetes mellitus.

Objectives:

1. Describe the pharmacologic therapy used for a patient with diabetes.
2. Evaluate a patient's response to insulin therapy.
3. Assess a patient for side effects of insulin therapy.
4. Describe the clinical manifestations of hypoglycemia as a side effect of insulin therapy.
5. Develop an individualized teaching plan for a patient with type 2 diabetes.

In this lesson you will learn the essentials regarding pharmacologic therapy for a patient admitted with complications related to diabetes mellitus. You will identify, describe, administer, and evaluate effects of prescribed antidiabetic medications. Harry George is a 54-year-old male with a 4-year history of type 2 diabetes admitted with infection and swelling of his left foot.

Exercise 1

 Clinical Preparation: Writing Activity

30 minutes

1. Identify and describe the various types of insulin by completing the table below.

Insulin Classification/ Generic Name	Brand Name	Onset (hour)	Peak (hour)	Duration (hour)
Rapid-Acting: aspart				
lispro				
glulisine				

Copyright © 2007 by Mosby, Inc., an affiliate of Elsevier Inc. All rights reserved.

Insulin Classification/ Generic Name	Brand Name	Onset (hour)	Peak (hour)	Duration (hour)
Short-Acting: regular insulin				
Intermediate-Acting: NPH				
lente				
Long-Acting: glargine				
determir				

2. Below, identify the five classifications of oral hypoglycemic agents, as well as specific medications and mechanism of action for each classification.

Classification	Medications	Mechanism of Action

3. Identify and describe two additional pharmacologic agents useful in treating diabetes mellitus.

Copyright © 2007 by Mosby, Inc., an affiliate of Elsevier Inc. All rights reserved.

Exercise 2

 CD-ROM Activity

 40 minutes

- Sign in to work at Pacific View Regional Hospital for Period of Care 1. (*Note:* If you are already in the virtual hospital from a previous exercise, click on **Leave the Floor** and then **Restart the Program** to get to the sign-in window.)
- From the Patient List, select Harry George (Room 401).
- Click on **Go to Nurses' Station**.
- Click on **Chart** and then **401**.
- Click on **Emergency Department**.

1. What medication was ordered to control Harry George's diabetes?

2. How would you give the IV insulin? (*Hint:* Consult the Drug Guide in the Nurses' Station.)

3. Look at the ED physician's progress notes for Monday at 1345. What does the physician plan to order for the sliding scale insulin coverage?

→ - Click on **Physician's Orders**.

4. Look at the orders for Monday at 1345. What was the actual sliding scale insulin order?

Copyright © 2007 by Mosby, Inc., an affiliate of Elsevier Inc. All rights reserved.

➡ • Click on **Return to Nurses' Station**.
  • Click on **Kardex** and then **401** for Harry George's record.

5. According to the Kardex, how often should the capillary blood glucose be tested?

➡ • Click on **Return to Nurses' Station**.
  • Click on **MAR** and then on tab **401**.

6. According to the MAR, when should the insulin sliding scale be administered? What was the time of this order?

7. What would you do regarding the inconsistencies identified above?

8. What problems might you anticipate for Harry George if he does not receive insulin coverage at bedtime?

➡ • Click on **Return to Nurses' Station** and then **401** to enter Harry George's room.
  • Click on **Clinical Alerts**.

9. What is the clinical alert for 0730?

Prepare and administer the sliding scale insulin for this glucose level by following these steps:

➡ • Click **Medication Room** on the bottom of the screen.
  • Click **MAR** or **Review MAR** at any time to verify how much insulin to administer based on sliding scale. (*Hint:* Remember to look at the patient's name on the MAR to make sure you have the correct records—you must click on correct room number within the MAR.) Click on **Return to Medication Room** after reviewing the correct MAR.

Copyright © 2007 by Mosby, Inc., an affiliate of Elsevier Inc. All rights reserved.

- Click on **Unit Dosage** and then on drawer **401** for Harry George's medications.
- Select **Insulin Regular**, click **Put Medication on Tray**, and then **Close Drawer**.
- Click **View Medication Room**.
- Click on **Preparation** and choose the correct medication to administer. Click **Prepare**.
- Click **Next**, choose the correct patient to administer this medication to, and click **Finish**.
- You can click on **Review Your Medications** and then **Return to Medication Room** when ready. Once you are back in the Medication Room, you can go directly to Harry George's room by clicking on **401** at the bottom of the screen.
- Click on **Patient Care**.
- Click on **Medication Administration** and follow the steps in the Administration Wizard to complete the insulin administration.

10. How much insulin should be administered?

11. What is the preferred site of administration for fastest absorption?

12. Fill in the chart below regarding the insulin you just administered.

	Expected Length of Time	Actual Time after 0730 Dose
Onset		
Peak		
Duration		

13. At what time would Harry George be most at risk for hypoglycemia? Describe the clinical manifestations that would indicate this acute complication.

14. While you are preparing to administer Harry George's insulin, he asks you why he is taking this since he did not use insulin at home. How would you answer him?

Copyright © 2007 by Mosby, Inc., an affiliate of Elsevier Inc. All rights reserved.

15. For what side effects should you monitor related to his insulin regimen?

Exercise 3

  CD-ROM Activity

40 minutes

- Sign in to work at Pacific View Regional Hospital for Period of Care 4. (*Note:* If you are already in the virtual hospital from a previous exercise, click on **Leave the Floor** and then **Restart the Program** to get to the sign-in window.)
- Click on **Chart** and then **401**. (*Remember:* You are not able to visit patients or administer medications during Period of Care 4. You are able to review patients' records only.)
- Click on **Nurse's Notes**.

1. Read the notes for Wednesday at 1730. What does Harry George request regarding glyburide?

2. How would you respond to the patient's demands?

3. How often did he take the glyburide at home?

4. Why do you think this was increased in the hospital? What concerns might you have regarding this increase? (*Hint:* Patient is also receiving insulin.)

Copyright © 2007 by Mosby, Inc., an affiliate of Elsevier Inc. All rights reserved.

5. What classification of oral hypoglycemics does glyburide belong to?

6. For what side effects of glyburide should you assess Harry George? (*Hint:* Click on the **Drug Guide** located on the counter in the Nurses' Station.)

7. What specific patient teaching points should you give this patient regarding glyburide?

8. What additional patient teaching related to diabetes would be appropriate for Harry George?

→ • Click on **Go to Nurses' Station**.
   • Click on **Chart** and then **401**.
   • Click on **Laboratory Reports**.

9. Chart Harry George's blood glucose and insulin administration since admission to the medical-surgical unit. (*Hint:* You may have to review the expired MARs in the chart to verify whether insulin was given for HS glucose measurement on Tuesday.)

Date/Time	Blood Glucose Level	Amount of Regular Insulin Administered

Copyright © 2007 by Mosby, Inc., an affiliate of Elsevier Inc. All rights reserved.

10. Based on Harry George's pattern of blood glucose levels, would you evaluate his current therapy as effective? If not, how might the physician further treat the patient's diabetes?

11. If you were reviewing the chart on Wednesday evening and found the information recorded in the table in question 9, what concern would you be ethically and legally bound to report?

Copyright © 2007 by Mosby, Inc., an affiliate of Elsevier Inc. All rights reserved.

LESSON **22** —————————————————————

Osteomyelitis

Reading Assignment: Nursing Management: Musculoskeletal Problems (Chapter 64)

Patient: Harry George, Room 401

Goal: Utilize the nursing process to competently care for patients with osteomyelitis.

Objectives:

1. Describe the pathophysiology of osteomyelitis.
2. Assess an assigned patient for clinical manifestations of osteomyelitis.
3. Describe the causative agent and category of osteomyelitis in an assigned patient.
4. Safely administer IV antibiotic therapy as prescribed for osteomylelitis.
5. Evaluate diagnostic tests related to osteomyelitis.
6. Develop an individualized discharge plan of care for a patient with osteomyelitis complicated by other disease processes and homelessness.

In this lesson you will learn the essentials of caring for a patient diagnosed with osteomyelitis. You will explore the patient's history, evaluate presenting symptoms and treatment, administer prescribed medications, and develop an individualized discharge teaching plan. Harry George is a 54-year-old male admitted with infection and swelling of his left foot, a history of type 2 diabetes, alcohol abuse, and nicotine addiction.

Exercise 1

 Clinical Preparation: Writing Activity

 10 minutes

1. Describe the pathophysiology of osteomyelitis.

Copyright © 2007 by Mosby, Inc., an affiliate of Elsevier Inc. All rights reserved.

2. Describe the two mechanisms of entry for pathogens causing osteomyelitis.

3. What is the most common causative organism of osteomyelitis?

Exercise 2

 CD-ROM Activity

 35 minutes

- Sign in to work at Pacific View Regional Hospital for Period of Care 2. (*Note:* If you are already in the virtual hospital from a previous exercise, click on **Leave the Floor** and then **Restart the Program** to get to the sign-in window.)
- From the Patient List, select Harry George (Room 401).
- Click on **Go to Nurses' Station**.
- Click on **Chart** and then **401**.
- Click on **History and Physical**.

1. The clinical manifestations of osteomyelitis can include both local and systemic symptoms. Common local and systemic signs and symptoms are listed below. Place an X next to any signs or symptoms consistent with Harry George's history and his physical examination findings on admission.

Local Symptoms	**Systemic Symptoms**
_____ a. Constant bone pain	_____ f. Fever
_____ b. Swelling	_____ g. Night sweats
_____ c. Tenderness	_____ h. Chills
_____ d. Warmth at infection site	_____ i. Restlessness
_____ e. Restricted movement	_____ j. Nausea
	_____ k. Malaise

Copyright © 2007 by Mosby, Inc., an affiliate of Elsevier Inc. All rights reserved.

2. What factors in Harry George's history may have contributed to the development of osteomyelitis? (*Hint:* See Table 64-1 in your textbook.)

3. Based on what you have read, identify the source of Harry George's osteomyelitis and the mechanism of invasion responsible for it. Explain the rationale for your conclusion.

 • Click on **Physician's Orders**.

 4. The following diagnostic tests are useful in the diagnosis and evaluation of osteomyelitis. Match each test with its corresponding description, as given in your textbook.

Diagnostic Test	**Description**
_____ MRI and CT scan	a. Initial test to determine causative organism
_____ Wound culture	b. Positive in the area of infection
_____ White blood cell count	c. Most definitive way to determine causative organism
_____ X-ray of affected extremitiy	
_____ Radionuclide bone scan	d. Elevated results of this test indicate infection
_____ Bone/tissue biopsy	e. Used to help identify the extent of the infection, including soft tissue involvement
_____ Erythrocyte sedimentation rate (ESR)	f. Changes with this test do not appear early in the course of the disease
	g. Elevated with inflammatory process

Copyright © 2007 by Mosby, Inc., an affiliate of Elsevier Inc. All rights reserved.

5. Place an X next to each diagnostic test that was performed as part of Harry George's admissions work-up.

_____ a. MRI and CT scan

_____ b. Wound culture

_____ c. White blood cell count

_____ d. X-ray of affected extremitiy

_____ e. Radionuclide bone scan

_____ f. Bone/tissue biopsy

_____ g. Erythrocyte sedimentation rate (ESR)

➡ • Click on **Diagnostic Reports**.

6. Compare the reports with the pathophysiology of osteomyelitis as described in your textbook. What findings documented on these reports are consistent with osteomyelitis? What do these findings mean?

Findings documented on the x-ray report

Findings documented on the bone scan

Meaning of both

➡ • Click on **Return to Nurses' Station**.
  • Click on **MAR** and select tab **401**.

Copyright © 2007 by Mosby, Inc., an affiliate of Elsevier Inc. All rights reserved.

7. Determine what routine medications (excluding the continuous IV and insulin coverage) you will be giving to Harry George during the day shift (0700-1500). Below, list the medications you need to give, the drug classification of each, the reason why each is given, and the time each is due. (*Hint:* You may refer to the Drug Guide by returning to the Nurses' Station and clicking on the **Drug** icon in the lower left corner of your screen.)

Medication	Classification	Reason for Giving	Time Due

8. Which medication was Harry George receiving that was discontinued on Tuesday?

→ • Click on **Return to Nurses' Station**.
  • Click on **Chart** and then **401**.
  • Click on **Physician's Orders**.

9. What replaced the medication you identified in question 8?

→ • Click on **Physician's Notes**.

10. Why was this change ordered?

→ • Click on **Laboratory Reports**.

Copyright © 2007 by Mosby, Inc., an affiliate of Elsevier Inc. All rights reserved.

11. You are aware that the antibiotics have been ordered for Harry George because of his leg infection. You decide to check the WBC results because you are curious (also, you are sure your nursing instructor will ask you about it). Document the WBC results for the times specified below and indicate whether each result is normal, elevated, or decreased.

Tests	Monday 1500	Tuesday 1100	Normal, Elevated, or Decreased?
Total WBC			
Neutrophil Segs			
Neutrophil Bands			
Lymphocytes			
Monocytes			
Eosinophils			
Basophils			

12. Explain what the WBC results in the table above mean, including the overall direction of the change in the WBC and the significance of this change.

➔ • Click on **Return to Nurses' Station**.
   • Click on **Patient List**.
   • Click on **Get Report** for Harry George. Review the report.

13. Is there anything else you wish the nurse would have included in the report regarding osteomyelitis? If so, what?

➔ • Click on **Return to Nurses' Station**.
   • Click on **Medication Room**.
   • Select **IV Storage**.
   • Click on the **Small Volume** bin and choose the IV antibiotic that is due to be given at 0800.

14. What dilution of this IV antibiotic is available for you to administer?

Copyright © 2007 by Mosby, Inc., an affiliate of Elsevier Inc. All rights reserved.

15. Over what amount of time should you infuse the IV antibiotic? (*Hint:* You may refer to the Drug Guide for this information.)

16. If you are using an IV pump to deliver this medication piggyback, what rate (mL per hour) will you select to give this infusion?

Exercise 3

  CD-ROM Activity

40 minutes

- Sign in to work at Pacific View Regional Hospital for Period of Care 2. (*Note:* If you are already in the virtual hospital from a previous exercise, click on **Leave the Floor** and then **Restart the Program** to get to the sign-in window.)
- From the Patient List, select Harry George (Room 401).
- Click on **Go to Nurses' Station** and then on **401**.
- Inside the patient's room, click on **Take Vital Signs**.

1. Record the vital sign findings below.

BP	SpO$_2$	Temp	HR	RR	Pain

- Click on **Patient Care**.
- Click on **Lower Extremities** and complete a focused neurovascular assessment related to osteomyelitis.

2. Below, record the results of your assessment.

- Click on **Patient Care** and then **Nurse-Client Interactions**.
- Select and view the video titled **1120: Wound Management**. (*Note:* Check the virtual clock to see whether enough time has elapsed. You can use the fast-forward feature to advance the time by 2-minute intervals if the video is not yet available. Then click on **Patient Care** and **Nurse-Client Interactions** to refresh the screen.)

Copyright © 2007 by Mosby, Inc., an affiliate of Elsevier Inc. All rights reserved.

3. How does the nurse describe the progress of Harry George's wound condition? How does the patient respond?

4. Based on your findings from questions 1 through 3, identify three priority nursing diagnoses for Harry George.

→ • Click on **Kardex**.

5. What interventions noted on the Kardex are related to Harry George's osteomyelitis?

→ • Click on **Medication Room**.
   • Click on **MAR** to determine what medications you need to administer to Harry George during this time period (1115-1200).
   • Click on **Return to Medication Room**.
   • Click on **IV Storage**.
   • Click on the **Small Volume** bin and choose the IV antibiotic that is due to be given at 1200.
   • Click **Put Medication on Tray**.
   • Click on **Close Bin**.
   • Click on **View Medication Room**.
   • Click on the **Drug** icon in the lower left corner of the screen.

6. Look up gentamicin in the Drug Guide. What must you assess prior to administering this drug? (*Hint:* Look at alert under Administration and Handling.)

Copyright © 2007 by Mosby, Inc., an affiliate of Elsevier Inc. All rights reserved.

→ • Click on **Return to Medication Room**.
  • Click on **Nurses' Station**.
  • Click on **Chart** and then **401**.
  • Click on **Laboratory Reports**.

7. What are Harry George's most recent peak and trough levels?

8. Based on these results, what should your nursing actions be?

9. For what toxic side effects must you monitor?

10. What types of follow-up diagnostic tests should be anticipated for Harry George to determine how well the osteomyelitis is responding to therapy? What changes will occur in these diagnostic test results if therapy is effective?

11. If Harry George's infection does not respond to the antibiotic therapy, what other interventions will most likely be planned? Explain how these would benefit him.

Copyright © 2007 by Mosby, Inc., an affiliate of Elsevier Inc. All rights reserved.

12. Based on what you know and have read, what do you expect will be included in Harry George's discharge instructions and follow-up care to manage his osteomyelitis?

13. Based on this patient's current living conditions, how do you think his care might best be managed?

Copyright © 2007 by Mosby, Inc., an affiliate of Elsevier Inc. All rights reserved.

LESSON 23

Chronic Low Back Pain

 Reading Assignment: Nursing Management: Musculoskeletal Problems (Chapter 64)

Patient: Jacquline Catanazaro, Room 402

Goal: Utilize the nursing process to competently care for a patient with an intervertebral disk problem.

Objectives:

1. Describe the pathophysiology of low back pain.
2. Identify clinical manifestations related to low back pain and/or herniated intervertebral disk.
3. Plan appropriate interventions to treat low back pain.
4. Evaluate a patient's potential to comply with a health care management plan.
5. Develop an individualized teaching plan for a patient with low back pain.

In this lesson you will learn the essentials of caring for a patient experiencing chronic low back pain. You will explore the patient's history, evaluate presenting symptoms and treatment, plan appropriate nursing interventions to treat the patient's symptoms, and develop an individualized discharge teaching plan. Jacquline Catanazaro is a 45-year-old female admitted with an acute exacerbation of asthma.

Exercise 1

Clinical Preparation: Writing Activity

15 minutes

1. List the risk factors for low back pain.

275

Copyright © 2007 by Mosby, Inc., an affiliate of Elsevier Inc. All rights reserved.

2. Identify five causes of low back pain.

3. Describe the pathophysiology of low back pain caused by degenerative disk disease.

4. What differentiates acute low back pain from chronic low back pain?

5. Describe the following procedures.

a. Intradiscal electrothermoplasty (IDET)

b. Radiofrequency discal nucleoplasty (coblation nucleoplasty)

c. Interspinous process decompression system (X STOP)

Copyright © 2007 by Mosby, Inc., an affiliate of Elsevier Inc. All rights reserved.

d. Laminectomy

e. Diskectomy

f. Microsurgical diskectomy

g. Percutaneous laser diskectomy

h. Charité disk implantation

i. Spinal fusion

Copyright © 2007 by Mosby, Inc., an affiliate of Elsevier Inc. All rights reserved.

Exercise 2

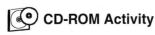 **CD-ROM Activity**

 45 minutes

- Sign in to work at Pacific View Regional Hospital for Period of Care 3. (*Note:* If you are already in the virtual hospital from a previous exercise, click on **Leave the Floor** and then **Restart the Program** to get to the sign-in window.)
- From the Patient List, select Jacquline Catanazaro (Room 402).
- Click on **Go to Nurses' Station**.
- Click on **Chart** and then **402**.
- Click on **History and Physical**.

1. Under "History of Present Illness," what are the patient's complaints related to her back?

2. How does the physician describe this problem under "Past Medical History"?

3. How was this diagnosed?

4. How long has the patient had this problem?

5. How would you classify Jacquline Catanazaro's back pain? Explain.

Copyright © 2007 by Mosby, Inc., an affiliate of Elsevier Inc. All rights reserved.

6. What treatment has she undergone? Explain the mechanism of action and/or rationale for these treatments.

➤ • Click on **Nursing Admission**.

7. What risk factors does Jacquline Catanazaro have for low back pain and/or degenerative disk disease?

8. What assessment should be completed on this patient in relation to the back pain?

➤ • Click on **Nurse's Notes**.

9. How have the nurses addressed Jacquline Catanazaro's complaint of low back pain?

Copyright © 2007 by Mosby, Inc., an affiliate of Elsevier Inc. All rights reserved.

10. What interventions could you suggest that would be appropriate for this patient's back pain during her hospital stay?

→ • Click on **History and Physical**.

11. What is the physician's plan regarding this patient's back pain? What type of interventions might be offered by this consult? (*Hint:* See Chapter 10 in your textbook for interventions.)

12. What formal program might be helpful for Jacquline Catanazaro? (*Hint:* See page 1676 in your textbook.)

13. What are the two goals for this program?

Copyright © 2007 by Mosby, Inc., an affiliate of Elsevier Inc. All rights reserved.

14. If her pain is not relieved by nonsurgical management, which of the procedures defined in your clinical preparation would you expect to be used for Jacquline Catanazaro? Why?

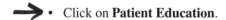 • Click on **Patient Education**.

15. What goals related to this patient's back pain would you add?

16. Develop a discharge teaching plan for Jacquline Catanazaro to help relieve and prevent further back pain.

Copyright © 2007 by Mosby, Inc., an affiliate of Elsevier Inc. All rights reserved.

• Click on **History and Physical**.

17. What may interfere with this patient's compliance to health care instructions?

 • Click on **Return to Nurses' Station**.
   • Click on **402** to enter Jacquline Catanazaro's room.
   • Click on **Patient Care** and then **Nurse-Client Interactions**.
   • Select and view the video titled **1540: Discharge Planning**. (*Note:* Check the virtual clock to see whether enough time has elapsed. You can use the fast-forward feature to advance the time by 2-minute intervals if the video is not yet available. Then click on **Patient Care** and **Nurse-Client Interactions** to refresh the screen.)

18. After viewing the video, what other suggestions do you have for assisting Jacquline Catanazaro with compliance after discharge? (*Hint:* Refer to Chapter 5 in your textbook.)

Copyright © 2007 by Mosby, Inc., an affiliate of Elsevier Inc. All rights reserved.

Osteoporosis

 Reading Assignment: Nursing Management: Musculoskeletal Problems (Chapter 64)

Patient: Patricia Newman, Room 406

Goal: Utilize the nursing process to competently care for patients with osteoporosis.

Objectives:

1. Describe the pathophysiology of osteoporosis.
2. Assess the assigned patient for clinical manifestations of osteoporosis.
3. Describe appropriate pharmacologic therapy for prevention and/or treatment of osteoporosis.
4. Describe the appropriate technique for safe administration of medications used to prevent or treat osteoporosis.
5. Plan appropriate interventions to promote health and prevent further bone loss in a patient with osteoporosis.
6. Develop an individualized teaching plan for an assigned patient with osteoporosis.

In this lesson you will learn the essentials of caring for a patient diagnosed with osteoporosis. You will explore the patient's history, evaluate presenting symptoms and treatment, administer prescribed medications, and develop an individualized discharge teaching plan. Patricia Newman is a 61-year-old female admitted with pneumonia and a history of emphysema.

Exercise 1

 Clinical Preparation: Writing Activity

10 minutes

1. Describe the pathophysiology of osteoporosis.

Copyright © 2007 by Mosby, Inc., an affiliate of Elsevier Inc. All rights reserved.

2. List the risk factors associated with osteoporosis.

Exercise 2

 CD-ROM Activity

 35 minutes

- Sign in to work at Pacific View Regional Hospital for Period of Care 2. (*Note:* If you are already in the virtual hospital from a previous exercise, click on **Leave the Floor** and then **Restart the Program** to get to the sign-in window.)
- From the Patient List, select Patricia Newman (Room 406).
- Click on **Go to Nurses' Station**.
- Click on **Chart** and then **406**.
- Click on **History and Physical**.

1. How long has Patricia Newman been diagnosed with osteoporosis?

2. What risk factors does she have for osteoporosis? Are any of these modifiable? If so, which ones?

3. What diagnostic test would have been ordered to diagnose this patient's osteoporosis? Describe the test and identify results diagnostic for osteoporosis.

Copyright © 2007 by Mosby, Inc., an affiliate of Elsevier Inc. All rights reserved.

➜ • Click on **Laboratory Reports**.

    4. Do any laboratory results for Patricia Newman correlate with osteoporosis?

➜ • Click on **Nursing Admission**.

    5. Are there any other risk factors found here?

    6. What clinical manifestation of osteoporosis is documented on this form?

    7. What other clinical manifestations would you assess Patricia Newman for in relation to osteoporosis?

➜ • Click on **Return to Nurses' Station**.
  • Click on **MAR** and select tab **406**.

Copyright © 2007 by Mosby, Inc., an affiliate of Elsevier Inc. All rights reserved.

8. What medications are ordered for Patricia Newman to help treat and prevent worsening of her osteoporosis? In the table below, identify these medications, their classifications, and mechanisms of action. You will complete the last column in question 9. (*Hint:* Consult the Drug Guide in the Nurses' Station.)

Medication	Drug Classification	Mechanism of Action	Side Effects

9. What side effects should you monitor Patricia Newman for related to these medications? Record your answer in column 4 of the table above.

10. If you were to administer the prescribed estradiol to this patient, how and where would you apply? Are there any precautions you should take while applying this?

Exercise 3

 CD-ROM Activity

 35 minutes

- Sign in to work at Pacific View Regional Hospital for Period of Care 3. (*Note:* If you are already in the virtual hospital from a previous exercise, click on **Leave the Floor** and then **Restart the Program** to get to the sign-in window.)
- From the Patient List, select Patricia Newman (Room 406).
- Click on **Go to Nurses' Station**.
- Click on **Chart** and then **406**.
- Click on **Patient Education**.

Copyright © 2007 by Mosby, Inc., an affiliate of Elsevier Inc. All rights reserved.

1. What educational goals already identified could be related to Patricia Newman's osteoporosis?

2. What teaching would you provide for Patricia Newman regarding exercise to prevent further bone loss?

3. What dietary needs does this patient have related to osteoporosis? What foods would you teach her to include in her diet?

4. What additional intervention to increase calcium absorption would you teach Patricia Newman?

Copyright © 2007 by Mosby, Inc., an affiliate of Elsevier Inc. All rights reserved.

5. Complete the following table to document teaching points you would review with Patricia Newman regarding her medications to treat osteoporosis.

Medication	Teaching Points

6. If Patricia Newman asked you what further treatment might be available to her if her bone loss continued despite her present regimen, how would you answer her? (*Hint:* Identify four other drug classifications that might be useful to this patient and describe their mechanism of action.)

7. What is Patricia Newman most at risk for related to her osteoporosis?

Copyright © 2007 by Mosby, Inc., an affiliate of Elsevier Inc. All rights reserved.

- Click on **Return to Nurses' Station** and then **406** to enter Patricia Newman's room.
- Click on **Patient Care** and then **Nurse-Client Interactions**.
- Select and view the video titled **1500: Discharge Planning**. (*Note:* Check the virtual clock to see whether enough time has elapsed. You can use the fast-forward feature to advance the time by 2-minute intervals if the video is not yet available. Then click on **Patient Care** and **Nurse-Client Interactions** to refresh the screen.)

8. Although the discussion in this video was related to the patient's pulmonary disease, how would smoking cessation benefit her musculoskeletal problem?

9. What other health care disciplines might be useful to help Patricia Newman with her discharge needs related to osteoporosis?

10. What psychosocial nursing diagnosis might be a potential problem for this patient related to her slightly stooped posture and going home on oxygen? What nursing interventions would be appropriate to help her with this difficulty?

Copyright © 2007 by Mosby, Inc., an affiliate of Elsevier Inc. All rights reserved.

LESSON 25

Osteoarthritis and Total Knee Replacement

Reading Assignment: Nursing Management: Musculoskeletal Trauma and Orthopedic
Surgery (Chapter 63)
Nursing Management: Arthritis and Connective Tissue Diseases
(Chapter 65)

Patient: Clarence Hughes, Room 404

Goal: Utilize the nursing process to competently care for patients with osteoarthritis.

Objectives:

1. Describe clinical manifestations and treatment for a patient with debilitating osteoarthritis.
2. Document a focused assessment on a postoperative patient who has undergone a total knee arthroplasty.
3. Plan appropriate interventions to prevent complications related to a total knee replacement in an assigned patient.
4. Identify and provide rationales for collaborative care measures used to treat a patient after a total knee arthroplasty.

In this lesson you will learn the essentials of caring for a patient undergoing a total knee arthroplasty for treatment of debilitating osteoarthritis. You will document assessments, plan, implement, and evaluate care given. Clarence Hughes is a 73-year-old male admitted for an elective knee replacement. Begin this lesson by reviewing the general concepts of osteoarthritis as presented in your textbook.

Exercise 1

Clinical Preparation: Writing Activity

10 minutes

1. Briefly describe the pathophysiology of osteoarthritis (OA).

Copyright © 2007 by Mosby, Inc., an affiliate of Elsevier Inc. All rights reserved.

2. List risk factors related to the occurrence of primary and/or secondary OA.

3. What are the clinical manifestations of OA?

4. What laboratory and/or radiographic testing are used in the diagnosis of OA?

Exercise 2

 CD-ROM Activity

40 minutes

- Sign in to work at Pacific View Regional Hospital for Period of Care 1. (*Note:* If you are already in the virtual hospital from a previous exercise, click on **Leave the Floor** and then **Restart the Program** to get to the sign-in window.)
- From the Patient List, select Clarence Hughes (Room 404).
- Click on **Go to Nurses' Station**.
- Click on **Chart** and then **404**.
- Click on **History and Physical**.

Copyright © 2007 by Mosby, Inc., an affiliate of Elsevier Inc. All rights reserved.

1. Why was Clarence Hughes admitted to the hospital?

2. Describe the symptoms that brought him to this point.

3. According to the H&P, what medications and/or treatments have been used to treat Clarence Hughes before he elected to have surgery?

4. According to your textbook, what is the usual indication for total knee arthroplasty?

→ • Click on **Surgical Reports**.

5. How does the report of operation describe the surgical procedure performed on Clarence Hughes?

6. What medication was added to the cement used for this procedure? Explain the rationale for the use of this medication.

Copyright © 2007 by Mosby, Inc., an affiliate of Elsevier Inc. All rights reserved.

7. What was Clarence Hughes' estimated blood loss (EBL)?

→   • Click on **Physician's Orders**.
    • Scroll down to read the orders for Sunday 1600.

8. What frequent assessments are ordered? Describe specifically how these assessments are completed and what the nurse is looking for.

→   • Scroll up to read the orders for Monday 0715.

9. What is ordered for Clarence Hughes' left knee? Explain the purpose of this machine.

📖 10. According to your textbook, what could be used to maintain extension of the operative knee?

→   • Click on **Return to Nurses' Station**.
    • Click on **EPR** and then on **Login**.
    • Select **404** as the patient and **Intake and Output** as the category.

11. Find "Output: Drain #1" for documentation of hemovac drainage. How much total drainage is recorded?

Copyright © 2007 by Mosby, Inc., an affiliate of Elsevier Inc. All rights reserved.

12. What were Clarence Hughes' I&O shift totals on Tuesday at 1500 and 2300?

 • Click on **Exit EPR**.
   • Click on **Chart** and then **404**.
   • Click on **Laboratory Reports**.

13. What was Clarence Hughes' H&H on Tuesday at 0600?

14. Why do you think his H&H was decreased? (*Hint:* Check his admitting H&H, EBL, drainage output, and 16-hour I&O on Tuesday.)

 • Click on **Physician's Orders**.

15. What was ordered to correct the above laboratory result?

Exercise 3

 CD-ROM Activity

45 minutes

• Sign in to work at Pacific View Regional Hospital for Period of Care 1. (*Note:* If you are already in the virtual hospital from a previous exercise, click on **Leave the Floor** and then **Restart the Program** to get to the sign-in window.)
• From the Patient List, select Clarence Hughes (Room 404).
• Click on **Get Report**.

Copyright © 2007 by Mosby, Inc., an affiliate of Elsevier Inc. All rights reserved.

1. What are your concerns for Clarence Hughes after receiving report?

→ • Click on **Go to Nurses' Station**.
   • Click on **404** to go to the patient's room.
   • Click on **Patient Care**.

2. Based on Clarence Hughes' diagnosis and surgery, complete a focused assessment and document your findings below.

Area Assessed	Findings
a.	
b.	
c.	
d.	
e.	

Copyright © 2007 by Mosby, Inc., an affiliate of Elsevier Inc. All rights reserved.

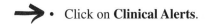 • Click on **Clinical Alerts**.

3. Based on these findings what would be your priority interventions?

 • Click on **Medication Room**.

- Click on **MAR** to determine prn medications that have been ordered for Clarence Hughes to address his constipation and pain. (*Note:* You may click on **Review MAR** at any time to verify the correct medication order. Remember to look at the patient's name on the MAR to make sure you have the correct record—you must click on the correct room number within the MAR. Click on **Return to Medication Room** after reviewing the correct MAR.)

- Click on **Unit Dosage** (or on the Unit Dosage cabinet); from the close-up view, click on drawer **404**.

- Select the medications you would like to administer. After each selection, click **Put Medication on Tray**. When you are finished selecting medications, click **Close Drawer**.

- Click on **View Medication Room**.

- Click on **Automated System** (or on the Automated System unit itself). Click **Login**.

- On the next screen, specify the correct patient and drawer location.

- Select the medication you would like to administer and click on **Put Medication on Tray**. Repeat this process if you wish to administer other medications from the Automated System.

- When you are finished, click **Close Drawer**. At the bottom right corner of the next screen, click on **View Medication Room**.

- From the Medication Room, click on **Preparation** (or on the preparation tray).

- From the list of medications on your tray, choose the correct medication to administer.

- Click **Next**, specify the correct patient to administer this medication to, and click **Finish**.

- Repeat the previous two steps until all medications that you want to administer are prepared.

- You can click on **Review Your Medications** and then on **Return to Medication Room** when ready. Once you are back in the Medication Room, you can go directly to Clarence Hughes' room by clicking on **404** at bottom of screen.

- Administer the medication, utilizing the five rights of medication administration. After you have collected the appropriate assessment data and are ready for administration, click **Patient Care** and then **Medication Administration**. Verify that the correct patient and medication(s) appear in the left-hand window. Then click the down arrow next to Select. From the drop-down menu, select **Administer** and complete the Administration Wizard by providing any information requested. When the Wizard stops asking for information, click **Administer to Patient**. Specify **Yes** when asked whether this administration should be recorded in the MAR. Finally, click **Finish**. You will evaluate your performance in this area at the end of this exercise (see question 14).

4. What is missing on the patient's order for oxycodone with acetaminophen? What measures need to be taken?

Copyright © 2007 by Mosby, Inc., an affiliate of Elsevier Inc. All rights reserved.

5. Based on the knowledge that most antacids frequently decrease absorption of other medications when concurrently administered, what options might the nurse employ to ensure adequate absorption of pain medication? (*Hint:* Consult the Drug Guide.)

 • Click on **Patient Care** and then **Nurse-Client Interactions**.
  • Select and view the video titled **0735: Empathy**. (*Note:* Check the virtual clock to see whether enough time has elapsed. You can use the fast-forward feature to advance the time by 2-minute intervals if the video is not yet available. Then click on **Patient Care** and **Nurse-Client Interactions** to refresh the screen.)

6. The nurse attempts to appear empathetic by offering to listen to the patient's concerns. Are her actions congruent with her verbal communication? Why or why not?

7. What would you as a student nurse do differently?

8. While planning nursing care for Clarence Hughes, identify five potential complications related to his postoperative status and measures that can be employed to prevent them. Document your plan of care below.

Complications   **Preventative Measures**

Copyright © 2007 by Mosby, Inc., an affiliate of Elsevier Inc. All rights reserved.

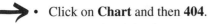 • Click on **Chart** and then **404**.
  • Click on **Consultations**.

9. What is physical therapy (PT) doing for Clarence Hughes?

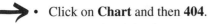 • Click on **Physician's Orders**.

10. What is the patient's activity order for Wednesday morning?

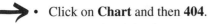 • Click on **Nurse's Notes**.

11. What is the patient's goal for CPM therapy today?

12. Do you think the ambulation and CPM goals are sufficient for the patient to be discharged tomorrow? Why or why not? (*Hint:* Look at his home situation in the nursing admission form.)

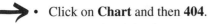 • Click on **Patient Education**.

13. What teaching should be completed for Clarence Hughes before his discharge?

Copyright © 2007 by Mosby, Inc., an affiliate of Elsevier Inc. All rights reserved.

Now let's see how you did during your earlier medication administration!

 • Click on **Leave the Floor** at the bottom of your screen.
- From the Floor Menu, select **Look at Your Preceptor's Evaluation**.
- Click on **Medication Scorecard**.

14. Disregard the report for the routine scheduled medications but note below whether or not you correctly administered the appropriate prn medications. If not, why do you think you were incorrect? According to Table C in this scorecard, what resources should be used and what important assessments should be completed before administering these medications? Did you utilize these resources and perform these assessments correctly?

Copyright © 2007 by Mosby, Inc., an affiliate of Elsevier Inc. All rights reserved.

Notes:

Notes: